beating
sports injuries

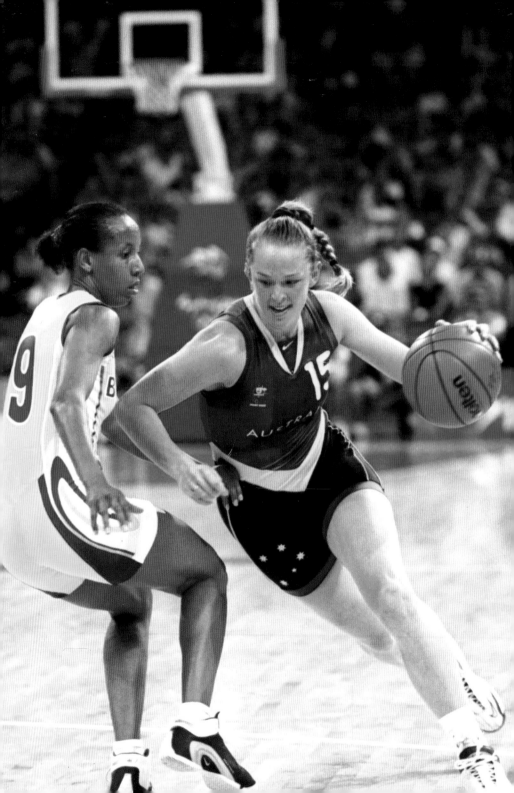

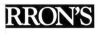 options for health

beating
sports injuries

Andrew Pallas

Dr. Len Saputo, Editor
Richard I. Gracer, M.D., Consultant

RRON'S

Beating Sports Injuries
Andrew Pallas

First edition for the United States and Canada published in 2002
by Barron's Educational Series, Inc.

All inquiries should be addressed to:
Barron's Educational Series, Inc.
250 Wireless Boulevard
Hauppauge, NY 11788
http://www.barronseduc.com

International Standard Book No.: 0-7641-1904-4

Library of Congress Catalogue Card No.: 2002100848

Additional titles in the *Options for Health* series:
Beating the Years
Boosting Your Digestive Health

Picture Credits
Front cover Stone/Henry Horenstein; 2 EMPICS Sports Photo Agency/Tony Marshall; 10
Corbis Stockmarket/LWA/Stephen Welstead; 13 SuperStock/Roger Allyn Lee; 21 Science
Photo Library/Peter Gardiner; 24 Corbis Stockmarket/Tom & Dee Ann McCarthy; 28 EMPICS
Sports Photo Agency/Jon Buckle; 33 SuperStock/Arlene Sandler; 37 Corbis Stockmarket/Jim
Cummins; 44 Corbis Stockmarket/Jim Cummins; 49 EMPICS Sports Photo Agency/Tony
Marshall; 57 SuperStock/Kwame Zikomo; 63 EMPICS Sports Photo Agency/Adam Davy;
69 EMPICS Sports Photo Agency/Mike Egerton; 73 SuperStock; 78 Photodisc; 82
SuperStock/Francisco Cruz; 87 Corbis; 89 EMPICS Sports Photo Agency/Tony Marshall; 95
SuperStock/Adam Smith; 105 EMPICS Sports Photo Agency/John Marsh; 107 Corbis/Jean
Pierre Lescourret; 109 Science Photo Library/Francoise Sauze; 118 SuperStock/Francisco
Cruz; 126 Stone/Erik Dreyer; 129 Photodisc; 135 Corbis/Ronnen Eshel; 137 Science Photo
Library/BSIP LECA; 139 Corbis Stockmarket/Rob Levine

Typeset in Futura and Folio
Printed and bound by Toppan Printing Company, China
9 8 7 6 5 4 3 2 1

contents

foreword

Most exercise-related injuries do not need to happen—they are preventable. However, when they do occur, it is important that you know what action to take. *Beating Sports Injuries* is an excellent resource that provides basic commonsense information that will help you minimize your risk of injury, understand the injury if it occurs, and manage it safely and wisely. It will help guide you to a speedy recovery, minimize possible complications, and facilitate your rehabilitation to optimal function through its user-friendly wisdom.

Andrew Pallas, M.D., has compiled accesible information derived from a wide variety of healthcare disciplines that collectively provide superior options for prevention and treatment. He skillfully guides you through every phase of managing your injury, whether you are a professional athlete or weekend warrior, so that you can remain active and healthy well into old age. His practical strategies can be individualized to meet your own needs and your own pace.

No single healthcare discipline has solved all of our health needs. However, it is possible to merge therapies from healthcare disciplines of conventional, alternative, and Eastern medicine to create innovative and powerful strategies designed to synergize your healing process. We live in an exciting and unique era that offers the miraculous technologies of modern medicine with the ancient wisdom of indigenous healing systems that have served humanity for thousands of years.

Pallas also addresses a deeper dimension that includes the whole person-body, mind, and spirit—as he explains why injuries occur and the myriad ways they can be managed. Attention to the psychology and meaning of sports is addressed, providing insights that can help you avoid injury and guide you to improve your skills as an athlete and your purpose as a human being. How you approach playing the "inner game" can make the difference that takes you to the next level of performance excellence in both sports and in the way you live your life. And, you will also likely find you will experience greater satisfaction and fun while you play.

Exercise is vital to ensure good health for everyone, but it is especially important for those with chronic degenerative diseases. There are many studies documenting that exercise improves the quality and the quantity of life in both the healthy and the ill. Increasing exercise to one hour a week for the couch potato carries with it significantly favorable outcomes. It is a kind of anti-aging "medicine" that keeps us young and helps prevent and treat many common health conditions. Modern scientific research has unequivocally documented that diseases, including cancer, strokes, diabetes, hypertension, osteoporosis, depression, anxiety, and even arthritis are less likely to affect those who are fit and active. And, if you do suffer from a chronic disease, the right exercise can promote healing and speed your restoration to good health.

The kind and intensity of exercise you choose should be tailored to your personal preferences, physical abilities, and lifestyle. In our busy high-tech lives, some of us fail to find time to include exercise. Once we get started, however, it can easily become the part of our day that we most enjoy. Practicing the exercise style that is right for you may be the key to avoiding injury, sustaining fitness, and feeling energized.

The United States government now officially recommends that we all get more exercise to ensure better health and reduce medical costs. It has become clear that the answer to the epidemic of chronic degenerative diseases we face in today's world resides in wellness and prevention rather than in treating diseases once they have occurred. Although there are many important lifestyle factors, such as diet, sleep, and stress reduction to consider, appropriate exercise may be the single most important factor that could make us less vulnerable to many of these illnesses.

It is not necessary to have the perfect physique or to be an Olympic athlete to enjoy sports. The form of exercise you choose can range from walking to distance running, and depends upon your abilities and preferences. Whatever form of exercise you choose, keeping in shape is likely to help you feel better and increase your longevity. And, the best part of all is that, through the right exercise, you'll have more fun, look younger, and enjoy better health and vitality throughout your life.

Dr. Len Saputo, Editor

introduction

In order to enjoy the healthy life we all crave, we are constantly being urged to make physical activity a part of our daily lives. It is well known that physical activity reduces the risk of many serious illnesses, including heart disease, strokes, obesity, and diabetes.

Significantly, sports can also add more fun to our lives. Research has demonstrated that physical activity is superior to relaxation techniques and equal to psychotherapy in combating depression. Enjoying a great workout is also a highly effective way of managing stress, so sports can be an important tool to help us cope with our ever-busier lives.

Risk of injury

Unfortunately, participating in sports also increases the risk of sustaining sports injuries. The effect of injuries goes beyond physical damage. They can also become sources of frustration and demoralization, as they may prevent us from participating in the sports we enjoy. The stress that is no longer relieved by the chosen activity is now compounded by the stress resulting from the injury. This can have long-term effects, as poorly managed injuries can recur once we resume activity, or become chronic conditions that persist, limiting our performance and enjoyment indefinitely.

However, the vast majority of sports injuries can be prevented. By developing an understanding of how injuries occur, you can take action to prevent them. The information contained in this book will help you continue to enjoy participating in sports, while minimizing the risk of injuries.

Coping with injury

The second purpose of this book is to help you decide what to do if you do sustain an injury. Huge amounts of money are spent on caring for expensive "elite" athletes, but how does the eager amateur best cope with injury, when resources and even sound advice are limited? You want to minimize time lost from sports, as well as from work and home activities. You want help to deal effectively with unpleasant symptoms, and you want to make a complete recovery and return to full fitness as quickly as possible. To do this, you need answers to the following questions:

- What has happened to my body?
- How can I help myself?
- What is the most appropriate professional treatment?
- How do I get back to fitness?

This book contains background information, such as how best to train or what safety measures to follow, along with information about injuries to a particular part of the body, such as the knee. You can also learn more about the different therapies that could help you.

Both conventional and complementary therapies are covered in this book, with information on self-treatment when appropriate. The best approach is to integrate a combination of methods that will support you in making a full recovery. You will also find guidance on those situations when you need to seek professional help.

How the tabs work

On the pages where specific injuries are discussed in part one are a series of colored tabs. These relate to the color-coded sections in part two of the book, guiding you to the therapies that are most likely to be useful for that injury, and where you will find more information on the suggested therapies.

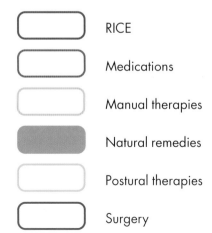

RICE

Medications

Manual therapies

Natural remedies

Postural therapies

Surgery

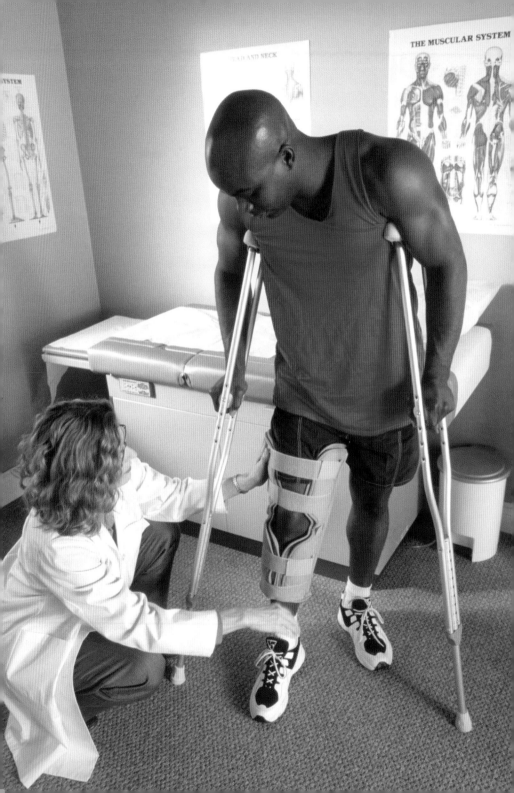

To understand your injury, you need a grasp of several basic concepts. You need to know how injuries occur, what the different tissues of your body do, and how stresses and strains can cause them to fail. This information is vitally important, because it allows you to choose appropriate training methods to prevent injuries. It also provides the basis for informed decisions about the care of any injury you do suffer.

The first section of this book covers all this for you, and cuts through the technical jargon that often accompanies information on healthcare.

UNDERSTANDING YOUR
sports injury

how
injuries
occur

The origin of some injuries is clear: such as in the boxer whose legs turn to jelly after a knock down, or the soccer player rolling round hugging one knee after a tackle. Yet many injuries occur for less obvious reasons.

You may feel sudden pain in your calf during a turn on the basketball court, or the breathtaking stab of back pain after an aerobics class. Such injuries are mysterious because you have made thousands of these moves before, and you had already finished the aerobic class. Other injuries come on more insidiously; the nagging groin pain that builds up over half a season, or the elbow pain that started as a mild ache when playing backhands in tennis and now stops you from picking up a briefcase.

Injuries are classed as either acute or chronic:
Acute refers to a condition that is short term, or a symptom that is sharp or sudden. A common cold is an acute illness – it is normally resolved over a few days. Similarly, a sprained ankle is an acute injury – it happens suddenly or sharply, and will often heal relatively quickly.

Chronic refers to conditions that persist over a long period of time. Arteriosclerosis or "hardening of the arteries" is a chronic condition, developing progressively over years. If you repeatedly re-sprain the same ankle, it could develop "chronic instability". Here, the ankle does not fully recover in the short term, and the resulting instability leaves it more vulnerable to further re-injury.

A too-common occurrence with sports injuries is that poor treatment and rehabilitation leaves the injured tissues weakened. Less able to stand up to normal stresses and strains, they are reinjured easily. The fact that many chronic sports injuries are the result of poorly managed acute injuries makes understanding injury prevention and treatment all the more important.

Acute injuries

Such injuries are often the result of **trauma**. This is usually caused by harmful contact, most commonly seen in contact sports such as boxing, football, rugby, and ice hockey. The contact need not be with another player, as traumatic injuries can also result from collisions with inanimate objects, like a squash player crashing into the court wall or the spectacular tumble of a downhill skier.

Acute strain is produced in several ways. First, the athlete exerts **excessive effort**—an effort that is greater than the tissues can cope with. An example of this could be an athlete training in a gym who tears a muscle by trying to lift too heavy a weight. Also in this category is the sprinter who "pulls a hamstring" while accelerating out of the blocks.

An Olympic champion gymnast or high jumper will make unbelievable feats appear almost effortless. This illusion is created, at least in part, by skills refined to the point that all

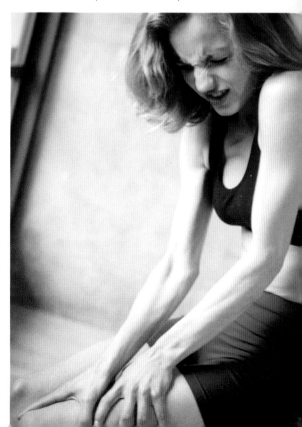

Pain while playing sports should always be taken as a sign to stop and assess the problem.

muscles work together to produce a smooth, coordinated movement. It is in the moments of incomplete coordination that injuries occur, when muscles work against each other, or produce inappropriate forces at joints.

Lack of warm-up commonly causes injury in recreational athletes. When the muscles and joints are unprepared, even low levels of stress can result in injuries.

Chronic injuries

As well as poorly treated or incompletely healed acute injuries, the other common type of chronic injury is that caused by prolonged inappropriate activity. These injuries can be exacerbated by biochemical deficiencies—for example, a tight ilutibial band combined with running may lead to chronic knee pain.

This damage is often undramatic, building up over a period of time before announcing itself with pain or restricted movement. We are blessed with natural self-repairing mechanisms, but continuous abuse can overcome these mechanisms. Abuse is broadly divided into **misuse** and **overuse**.

Misuse

Misuse can stem from **poor technique** and **preexisting problems**.

Poor technique is a common source of injury in recreational and amateur athletes. Poor technique may concentrate stress onto specific areas of the body. For example, jogging on the balls of the feet, rather than landing naturally on the heels, produces undue strain on the ankle, foot, Achilles tendon, and calf muscles.

To avoid these problems, learn good techniques for your sport and constantly refine them. Working with a qualified coach is useful for even the most experienced athlete. But be careful of the less expert advice of other athletes. They may be well informed or they may not be, even if they speak with great confidence.

Preexisting problems from years of working hunched over a computer can cause a stooped posture with the shoulders forward and a bowed upper back. Imagine someone with such a stooped posture taking up a racket sport, where overhand strokes demand the arm to be raised up vertically or beyond. The stiff back could result in exaggerated strains on the shoulder because it is performing its own function, plus undertaking the work that should have been done by the upper back bending backward slightly. Hence a "normal" motion may, over time, cause injury to the shoulder.

If you have any physical impairment or disability, make sure that all techniques and equipment are adapted to suit you. This is likely to need specialist advice. See the list of organizations on p.141 for sources of help. Remember that the techniques and equipment are there to serve you, not the other way around.

Overuse

The most obvious cause of overuse injuries is **overtraining**. This is a particular risk when people embark on a new sport or activity. Enthusiasm often drives us to do more than we safely can. Look for excesses in training frequency, duration, intensity, or any combination of these factors. To prevent these injuries, develop a plan to gradually build up your fitness and level of training. Monitor your response so that you can reduce your training load if necessary. An unrealistic attitude to training can lead to injury. By competing within your capacity and by focusing on your achievements rather than those of your teammates or opponents, you can avoid injury and also increase your ability to participate effectively. For more advice see the section on training principles beginning on p.88.

The other key danger point for overtraining is when athletes reach plateaus in their progress. Many fall into the trap of thinking that because training is good, then more training must be better. Chronic overtraining results in diminished performance, fatigue, a reduction in enthusiasm, and an increased risk of injury. Cope with plateaus by improving the quality rather than the quantity of your training. This is another situation where the advice of a good coach can be invaluable.

An easily missed cause of overtraining is when training and other aspects of your life combine to produce the effects of overtraining. Are you a long-distance runner who already covers five miles a day as a postal worker, or a weight lifter working for a removal firm all day? If your occupation is physically demanding, moderate your training program accordingly, ensuring that you are allowing sufficient recovery time between sessions.

the **healing process**

If you suffer an injury, the choices you make about what to do next can have a major impact on your recovery. Information alone is not enough to help you make wise choices – you need to understand enough to apply the correct principles to your own situation. This section explains the fundamentals of the healing process, so that you can make educated decisions to speed your recovery.

What makes healing happen?

It is important to remember that healing is perfectly natural and happens by itself. No treatment will heal your injury – you heal your injury yourself. The purpose of treatments is to remove obstacles to that healing. Such obstacles can impair the normal healing response, reducing its effectiveness, slowing it down, or even stopping it completely.

A whole host of mechanisms throughout the body and mind have to work adequately for healing to occur, so even obstacles that seem to have nothing to do with your injury can still influence your recovery. Let's look at a "simple" example like a sprained ankle that is refusing to settle in order to explore this further.

■ If the fall or twist that injured the ankle also strained your hip or lower back, the alteration in the way you walk caused by these strains may be stressing your ankle, preventing it from settling. Despite this, you may not have any symptoms in your hip or lower back.

■ The ankle ligament can only repair itself if the necessary raw materials are available. Any nutritional imbalance may slow the healing process. The body needs protein in order to rebuild the new ligament but much of this may come from the body's ability to "recycle" the old damaged ligament. Several "micronutrients" such as vitamin C, the mineral manganese, and glucosamine sulphate (see p.127), are required to rebuild ligaments properly.

■ If, as is very common, your diet is high in fats, there can be an excessive accumulation of their breakdown products, called ketone bodies, in the body, which are highly acidic, and can increase inflammation and impede the healing process. It is important to include some fats in your diet, but they should provide no more than 30 to 35 percent of your total calories (according to the American Heart Association). High levels of saturated fats, as found in meat and dairy foods, or highly processed fats, such as in many snack foods, are "bad" fats. Healthier options include monounsaturated fats, such as olive oil, canola oil, and avocados. Essential fatty acids (EFAs) are used to produce hormones that are vital mediators in the inflammatory process, but the wrong kind of fats can have adverse effects on this. This may mean that the inflammatory phase of the healing process may not resolve itself. This is one cause of "chronic inflammation," which leads to stubborn injuries that can pose a real challenge to treatment.

■ Several kinds of belief can actually impair your ability to heal yourself. If you accept the erroneous idea, for example, that you should "work the pain off," you will continue to redamage your ankle, and your healing will take one step forward and two back. Or perhaps you get depressed by your inability to participate in your usual sport. Because such low states influence the balance of hormones within your body, they can literally "depress" your body's ability to recover from injuries or illnesses. This can establish a vicious cycle with injury causing depression, and depression maintaining injury.

How healing happens

If a storm tore part of the roof and a section of wall off your house, there is a definite process you would have to go through to deal with the damage. You would need some tarpaulin to protect your possessions from the weather. Gas and water supplies would need to be turned off, in case leaks caused further damage.

Next you would want contractors to come and start repairing the damage by replacing lost or damaged parts of your house with new ones. For this, they would need deliveries of the required materials. Some damage would probably be repaired using different materials from the original. For instance, minor cracks in brickwork might be repaired with fillers rather than with bricks and mortar.

The process of healing damaged tissues is, in many respects, very similar. One of the first responses to injury is the constriction of damaged blood vessels. This is like turning off the gas and water supplies, and it aids the formation of a blood clot or "scab," which stems blood loss. In addition, if the injury is exposed to the outside world, the scab protects us against infection by microorganisms. The scab is our very own tarpaulin. But just because there is no break in the skin, this doesn't mean that blood is not being lost. Blood lost from the circulation can pool under the skin, producing a bruise, or leak into muscle, joints, or body cavities.

Inflammation

The next step in the healing process is the inflammatory response. This dilates blood vessels in the area, which increases blood flow to the area, causing redness and heat as a result. Again, it is important to remember that just because there is no break in the skin, it does not mean that blood is not being lost.

Inflammation results in the blood vessels in the injured area becoming more permeable. This allows our defensive army of white blood cells into the injury site, so that they can digest any invading bacteria, along with the debris from damaged tissues. Leaking out of the blood vessels is fibrin—a sticky material used to temporarily "shore up" the damaged tissue, and to further impede the spread of any bacteria.

Inflammation is easy to spot if the injury site is near the surface of the body—a sprained ankle is a familiar example. The area becomes **hot** and **red** because of the increased blood supply around the injury (only the damaged blood vessels within the injury site itself constrict), and the leaking of fluid into the surrounding tissues produces **swelling**. Chemicals released from the damaged tissue, and by the inflammatory reaction itself, irritate nerves, which causes pain.

Proliferation

At this stage of the healing process, cells replicate to rebuild the tissue as much as possible—the equivalent of the contractors beginning to rebuild your wall and roof. Sometimes not all of the damaged tissue is replaced with new tissue, but is replaced by a scar instead. This is like the contractors' silicone filler—it is adequate, but not quite as good as the original tissue. One aspect of effective treatment is to reduce the amount of scar tissue being formed by creating the conditions that allow the body to generate replacement tissue. Scar tissue tends to be formed if there is inadequate oxygen supply in the area to sustain more active tissue. This is why, once bleeding has stopped, treatments that encourage circulation into the injury site are beneficial.

This is called the stage of proliferation because tissue increases or proliferates, sometimes beyond what was there originally. At this stage, for example, the repair to a broken bone is thicker than the original bone. The injury is now apparently healed but will not yet be back to full strength. This is a critical time in the rehabilitation process, as it is easy to overstress the new tissue, causing reinjury.

Remodelling

At this stage the new tissue is remodelled so that it regains its functional strength. The modelling process is guided by the stresses imposed on the new tissue, with fibers lining up to withstand the loads applied to them. This is similar to what happens if you start to train with weights. Your muscles build up to withstand the stresses you apply to them; the result is that you remodel yourself.

This is why injuries that are only rested for a short while often reinjure with the return to activity. The new tissue is there, but it has not built up its strength, so, as soon as it is loaded again, it fails. The progressive rehabilitation of tissues, to return them to functional strength, is an essential and often overlooked part of dealing with sports injuries. For more information, see the section on rehabilitation beginning on p.138.

Overcoming obstacles to healing

There are often several factors involved in any injury, which means there are various ways in which you can help yourself back to fitness. To optimize your healing capability, address as many aspects as possible that can influence it.

It is not necessary to remove every little obstacle for healing to occur, as your natural healing mechanisms will climb over any obstacle they can. However, making their job easier is obviously in your best interest.

We don't yet know all the answers, but by acting on the information in this book, you will give yourself a wide range of options to help your body heal itself.

identifying
your
problem

To choose appropriate treatment, you have to know what
the problem is. Recognizing when a tissue is no longer
functioning normally requires you to know what it does
normally. This section contains information about the different
tissues, and how you might identify which ones are injured.

The diagram opposite illustrates a typical joint, and the functions of each of the
different tissues are listed below.

Skin

Skin is our outer barrier, separating our internal and external environments. It
protects us from infection by stopping bugs coming in, and it protects us from
dehydration by stopping water leaking out. It is our largest organ of excretion,
eliminating wastes in sweat, which also doubles as a cooling mechanism,
preventing us from overheating. Skin can be damaged by trauma, producing cuts
(lacerations) or grazes (abrasions). It can also suffer from infection, such as "athlete's
foot". Outdoor sports can expose skin to sunburn and stings from plants or insects.

Fascia

This tissue is vital to the mechanical and functional integrity of the body. Fascia links
together all of the components of the body and carries nerves, blood, and lymphatic
vessels through it. Skeletal muscles are covered and held together by fascia, which
protects them and provides attachment points to bones and other muscles via

tendons. In this way, fascia acts to carry and distribute the weight of the body during movements. For example, the "plantar fascia" in the foot helps to hold up the arches when standing, walking, or running.

Muscles and tendons

Muscles are our engines, turning the energy released from food into movement. They produce heat, which is why exercise makes us warm, and also produce waste. This has to be removed by our circulation, otherwise it builds up and causes fatigue, stiffness, and sometimes pain.

Muscles work by contracting (where they get shorter). So muscles can only pull, they can't push. To enable us to do both pushing and pulling movements, muscles are arranged in opposing pairs or groups. For instance, the muscle at the front of your upper arm, the biceps, bends your elbow, while the muscle at the back of your arm, the triceps, straightens your elbow.

Tendons are responsible for connecting muscles to the bones they move—they are the ropes that the muscles pull on. Tendons don't do active work, so they need

The elements of a typical joint

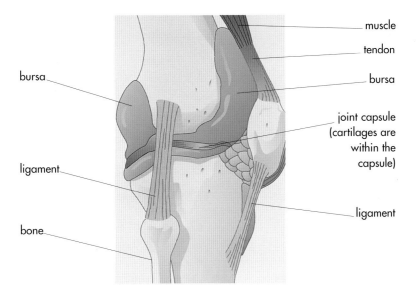

muscle

tendon

bursa

bursa

joint capsule (cartilages are within the capsule)

ligament

ligament

bone

much less blood supply than muscles, but this does mean an injured tendon is usually slower to heal.

An injury to a muscle or tendon may be a complete rupture, where it is torn in two; but, more typically, only some of the fibers are torn. When a muscle–tendon unit is injured, asking it to work against resistance is painful. Where the tear is near the surface, bleeding from it may produce visible bruising.

Bone

Bones are stiffening rods, like a tent's poles, that allow us to stand up. They are also the levers that muscles pull on in order to produce movement. Some bones, like the skull and ribs, protect delicate internal organs. Blood cells are produced in the core of long bones (such as the main bones in the arms and legs), and bone also acts as a store for calcium, which is needed for activities such as muscular contraction.

Bones are relatively stiff, so injured bones may break or "fracture." A fracture produces swelling, and pain that is aggravated by movement. An "avulsion" fracture occurs when the contraction of a muscle is so strong that it pulls off part of the bone where its tendon is attached.

Most fractures require immobilization, often with a cast, to allow healing. Occasionally, fractures are complicated, and therefore require surgery to pin or plate pieces together.

Joints

Joints are the meeting points of two or more bones, and allow bones to move relative to each other. The components of a "typical" joint include:

Ligaments These are the straps that tie bones together at a joint, adding stability. They can be damaged by forces acting against the joint. For example, ligaments help stabilize the knee against bending sideways, so forces that push the knee sideways, if strong enough, will damage the ligaments. Injured ligaments cause pain and swelling around the joint, and overstretched ligaments may lead to joint instability.

If ligaments are torn completely, the joint may move in abnormal directions. The more common partial tears can quite quickly allow pain-free movement, so long as the movement is not in a direction that stresses the ligament. However, like tendons, ligaments have poor blood supplies and so they heal slowly. Therefore, it is very important to ensure that you do not overuse them too soon after an injury. Just because you don't feel pain in the area does not mean it has healed completely, so you must give it time to recover fully.

Cartilage The ends of bones within a joint are covered in cartilage, providing a smooth and slightly shock-absorbent surface. Damage to this cartilage can make the joint more susceptible to wear. Some joints have additional cartilages that act like washers, filling in spaces between bones that do not fit exactly. Examples include the cartilages within the knee and the jaw joints.

Joint capsule This is a specialized kind of ligament. It forms a bag around the joint to contain the lubricating fluid known as synovial fluid. The capsule is lined with synovial membrane, which produces the synovial fluid, so our joints are self-lubricating. The joint capsule can be injured in the same way as ligaments.

Bursa These are fluid-filled sacks that are positioned at certain points around some joints. They act as cushions, separating and padding adjacent tissues. High levels of stress on an area can cause the bursa to become inflamed and swollen, a condition known as a "bursitis." In "housemaid's knee," for example, prolonged kneeling causes the bursa at the front of the knee to become painful and swollen.

Nerves

Nerves carry information from one part of the body to another. They carry orders from the brain out to the body, allowing you to run, throw, or wiggle your toes when you want to. Nerves also report information from muscles and joints, so that our brain knows what is going on and can coordinate our movements.

Pain messages from damaged tissues tell us that damage has occurred and warn us if we do anything to make the situation worse. Injuries that damage the nerves alter the information coming in, resulting in numbness ("pins and needles"), or alter the information going out, resulting in difficulty or inability to contract muscles. Problems with the autonomic nervous system, which controls the subconscious functions of the body, such as heart rate, can also cause abnormal blood supply and delay healing.

when to seek
professional
advice

There are several circumstances that can arise as a result of sustaining an injury when you should seek professional advice. Some situations, such as a broken bone, require immediate attention and should be dealt with in the emergency department of a hospital. Others, such as an ankle sprain that is not healing adequately, can wait for an appointment with a healthcare professional.

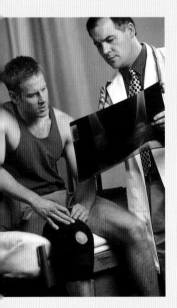

In the latter instance, the next thing you need to consider is which health professional to see. Refer to the information on specific injuries in the following sections, to try and identify your injury. The colour-coded tabs will also guide you to which professions you might wish to consult.

If you are not able to identify your injury, then it would be wise to consult a practitioner who is qualified as a primary care provider, such as a medical practitioner with an interest in sports injuries (for example an orthopaedic physician, an osteopath, or a chiropractor). Details of the different professions are provided in Part Two: All the Options.

If you are in any doubt about your injury, seek professional advice.

This includes all incidents or injuries that are in the warning boxes throughout the book, plus any that cause:

- *A loss of consciousness or persistent headache, nausea, vomiting, or dizziness.*
- *Sustained difficulty breathing (beyond having the "wind knocked out of you").*
- *Persistent chest pain.*
- *Neck pain from an impact.*
- *Signs that cause you to suspect a fracture, dislocation, or severe joint injury.*
- *Signs of a muscle or tendon tear.*
- *Blood loss that is not easily controlled.*
- *Significant skin damage, such as a deep cut, in which stitches may be required.*
- *Any eye injury.*
- *Any injury you are not sure about (better to be safe than sorry).*

Any severe or persistent injury to a child or adolescent should be professionally evaluated. This is because their bodies are not yet fully developed, so any injury could cause permanent damage.

Where emergency treatment may be needed, do not have anything to eat or drink, in case a general anaesthetic is required.

Problems that require professional advice

- Any injury where you are uncertain of the diagnosis.
- Any injury that does not heal as expected.

Symptoms of general health problems should never be passed off as being the result of a sports injury. Injuries that occur because of sports activities do not cause fevers, night sweats, abdominal pain, shortness of breath, or pain that is constant despite changes of activity or position. In all such cases, you should seek the advice of your healthcare provider.

INJURIES

This part of the book covers specific injuries, and is divided into sections for each area of the body. Each one gives information on injuries that are common, or serious enough that you should be aware of them. For each injury you will find:

- A description of the injury
- Likely ways the injury could occur
- What you might see or feel if you had the injury
- Where applicable, what self-treatment you could use
- What professional treatment options would be helpful

from head to toe

Getting the right treatment

On the pages dealing with each injury, you will find colored tabs that refer you to the color-coded sections in Part Two: Options for Health. This indicates the therapies that would be appropriate to consider for treatment. Injuries discussed in the warning boxes (the grey boxes with an exclamation mark) require emergency medical or surgical attention. If you suspect one of these injuries in yourself or others, you should arrange for immediate transport to the nearest hospital that provides emergency treatment.

In Part Two: Options for Health, you can find information about ways of preventing injuries, as well as a variety of therapies useful in the treatment and rehabilitation of injuries. To help you locate practitioners in your area, contact details of appropriate organizations are given on p.141.

For clarity, each injury is discussed as if it were a discrete, separate problem. In reality, injuries often have several aspects to them that need to be considered. The fact that someone can diagnose a muscle strain of the lower back, for example, does not rule out the possibility of a sprained spinal joint or weak abdominal muscles as well.

We start this section with information on injuries to the head, face, and neck. These chapters begin with details of the most serious injuries of all, not because they are common, but because appropriate initial care is so important. Thankfully, even professionals providing athletic healthcare don't see these injuries too frequently.

Complementary therapies

While giving appropriate attention to the immediate area of an injury is important, it is equally important to see the injury as the final point of breakdown in you as a whole. It is your whole being that must recover, and you as a whole whose approach to sports will help to prevent further injuries.

Refer to Options for Health for the complementary treatment options that will support your natural healing mechanisms. Recovery from an injury could be speeded up by using appropriate nutrition and hydrotherapy, along with herbal or homeopathic remedies. The more ways you can support and encourage your natural healing mechanisms, the more rapid your return to full fitness is likely to be.

head
and face
injuries

While head injuries can be very serious, even fairly minor injuries to the head can be upsetting. Potentially dangerous injuries that need emergency medical assessment include fractures, injuries causing impairment of consciousness, and injuries affecting the function of the eye or ear.

Any blow that causes a loss of consciousness, however short, should result in the victim being taken to an emergency department. Always accompany them to the hospital and, if possible, give a description of the incident to the attending doctor.

Other serious symptoms following a head injury are dizziness, nausea or vomiting, and mood changes. While these types of head injuries are not particularly common sports injuries, they have been included here because of their seriousness.

Head injuries require careful evaluation.

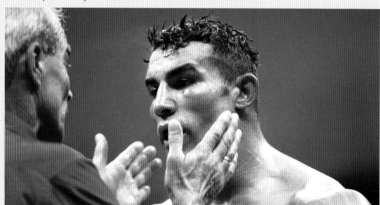

FRACTURES

Fractures are usually the result of a blow or collision, and so are more likely to occur in contact or collision sports, such as football, boxing, or rugby. The bones of the skull, face, or jaw may all be affected. If the person is conscious, pain is likely to be a prominent symptom. Other signs of skull fractures are:

- *Blood or a clear, straw-colored fluid leaking from the nose, eyes, or ears.*
- *Bruising behind the ear or around the eyes (known as the "Panda sign").*

Fractures of the facial bones can cause:
- *Eye movements to be painful.*
- *The pupils of the eyes to be at different heights.*
- *Double vision.*
- *A numb cheek.*

Jaw bone fractures can lead to:
- *Pain when attempting to open the mouth or clench the teeth.*
- *The teeth being misaligned. They look or feel as if they are not meeting normally when the mouth is closed.*

In all cases where you suspect a fracture, go directly to the nearest hospital that has an emergency room. The victim should not be given anything to eat or drink, in case an anaesthetic is required. Help to reduce pain and bleeding by the gentle application of an ice pack to the area. Wrap the ice pack in something like a T-shirt before applying it, as you should never apply ice directly to the skin due to the risk of ice burns. An ice pack over the eye should only be left on for five minutes maximum, to prevent the risk of damage to the eye itself.

The pain of a fractured jaw can often be reduced by supporting the jaw with a bandage or scarf, which should go under the jaw and be knotted on the top of the head. The reduction in discomfort should be your guide to ensuring it is neither too tight nor too loose. This should help reduce pain as you travel to the hospital.

Nose injury

Nosebleeds are a fairly common problem, and are usually the result of an impact. To deal with a simple nosebleed:

- Lean the head forward, and pinch the nose about halfway down, just below the end of the nose bone. (Leaning back causes blood to go down the throat.)
- To help control the bleeding, use ice over the nose or on the base of the neck. This causes blood vessels to constrict or narrow, slowing the flow.
- Check in a mirror. If the nose is deviated, suspect a fracture and go to the hospital. A broken nose is not usually a serious injury, but realignment, to maintain your appearance and ease of breathing, is much easier if done early on.

Eye injuries

Grit, mud, or other foreign bodies in the eye should be initially treated by washing the eye with clean, running water. Make sure you wash **away from the nose**, otherwise you could wash the object out of one eye and into the other. You will probably need to hold your eyelids open with your fingers to allow the water in. If the foreign body is not removed by washing, go to the hospital. If eye movements cause pain, cover both eyes as this prevents unnecessary movements.

Blows to the area around the eye can produce the bruising of a "black eye." Treat this with an ice pack as soon after the injury as possible. Remember that the ice pack should not be in contact with the eye itself for more than five minutes at a time. See natural remedies beginning on p.128 for more ways to treat bruising.

Blows to the eye can cause a "blow-out" fracture, where bones within the eye socket are damaged. If there are any signs of fracture (see facial fractures on p.29) or if vision becomes blurred as a result of an injury, a hospital visit is required.

Ear injuries

The ears are primarily affected by cuts or friction. Treat minor cuts by cleaning and dressing them with a plaster or bandage; cuts to the ears are no exception. Bleeding from deeper cuts can often be controlled by direct pressure and an ice pack over the area. Instances where bleeding is difficult to control, or where cuts are deep, should be checked in a hospital in case stitches (suturing) are required.

A "Cauliflower Ear" is a swelling produced by bleeding into the substance of the ear. It is usually caused by friction or a blow. An ice pack will slow the bleeding. A doctor may drain the blood with a syringe (aspiration) to prevent the development of a chronic deformity. Damage to the ear drum from loud noises, such as gunfire in shooting events, or from pressure while diving will impair hearing. Once again a hospital visit is required. Swimmers can suffer infections of the ear, resulting in irritation and redness. Orthodox medical treatment uses antibiotic drops, for which you could substitute a light carrier oil, such as almond oil, mixed with tea tree oil.

DENTAL INJURIES

Teeth being knocked out is common in contact sports. Knowing the appropriate action to take can save a tooth. If a tooth is knocked out, and no other more serious injury is suspected, you should:

- *Place a wad of cotton wool into the tooth socket, and bite on it lightly to control the bleeding.*
- *Keep the tooth damp, preferably in sterile saline, milk, or the person's own saliva.*
- *Leave the tooth as is.*
- *Get to a dentist within 30 minutes to greatly increase the chances of the tooth being successfully reimplanted.*

neck
injuries

Neck injuries range from the minor to the catastrophic. Neck injuries are common but thankfully the really serious injuries are not. The worst-case scenario is the neck fracture.

Neck strains

Most people have experienced minor neck strain at one time or another. For example, turning your head quickly can cause an instant burning sensation in your

---

NECK FRACTURES

Fractures are usually of traumatic origin, most likely in contact sports or in sports where falls onto the head can occur, particularly equestrian events. Indications of a neck fracture are:
- *The injury involved trauma to the head or neck.*
- *A conscious person is unable to move one or more of their limbs, or is unable to feel you touching their limbs.*
- *If the person is unconscious, it will be difficult to get any other clues, so assume a fracture until you know otherwise.*

In such instances, do not move them until medical assistance arrives. The only exceptions to this rule are:
- *If they have stopped breathing, in which case turn them onto their back so that CPR (Cardio Pulmonary Resuscitation) can be performed.*
- *The surroundings pose a serious threat to life (for example, a burning car in a motor sport event).*

If at all possible get help so that you can keep their head and body in line (both facing the same direction) while you turn them.

---

neck, usually on the side you are turning away from. The strain involves a tearing of some of the fibers of a muscle, and may be associated with spasm of the muscle. Both will produce pain when the muscle is stretched. A tear will also be painful if you contract the muscle against resistance. If turning your head to the right causes pain and attempting to turn your head to the left against resistance also causes pain, then you have probably strained a muscle.

Likely causes of neck strains include intense effort against resistance, among wrestlers or judo competitors, or, more commonly, sudden uncoordinated movements of the head in any sport. Strains are more likely if the muscle is cold or lacks flexibility.

Initial treatment is rest and the application of ice. If the strain is minor, gently maintain mobility by slowly moving your head within pain-free limits. Non-steroidal Anti-Inflammatory Drugs (NSAIDs) may be prescribed for symptomatic relief, but the acidic content of these drugs can cause side effects, such as indigestion and nausea (see p.106). Complementary therapies such as nutrition (see p.124), acupuncture (see p.120), homeopathy, and natural remedies (see p.128) are good alternatives.

If the pain and restricted movement persist, you should seek professional advice from a manual therapist. He may provide manual treatment to relax spasm and speed healing, prescribe exercises, or use some form of electrotherapy.

The location of pain may not be the site of the injury, but it provides useful clues.

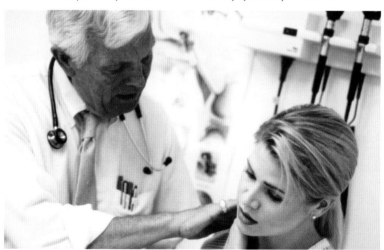

Joint sprain or dysfunction

The same stresses that cause neck muscle strain can also cause problems for the joints in the neck. A sprain involves tearing of the fibers in ligaments around a joint.

Movement of any body part requires the coordinated action of many components. Lack of this coordination can result in a "stuck" joint and deep muscle spasm. The joint becomes "dysfunctional," even if tissues are not damaged.

The symptoms are similar to neck strain, with one or more movements being limited and painful. Another symptom can be displaced pain, which may be felt at the back of the head, across the shoulder, or down the arm. Tingling or pins and needles may also be present in the same areas. If displaced symptoms persist for more than a few minutes, seek a professional assessment.

Initial treatment is the application of ice and plenty of rest, with gentle movement within the pain-free range to maintain mobility. NSAIDs are often supplied for this, but current evidence suggests the anti-inflammatory effect of these drugs is minimal in such cases. Natural remedies can provide effective symptomatic relief.

A practitioner will search for the cause of the symptoms, which could be in the joints of the upper back as well as the neck. Treatment will be aimed at relaxing the spasm, thus restoring normal blood flow to the area and regaining normal mobility in the joint. Methods are described in manual therapies, beginning on p.108.

Trapped nerve

We have already touched on the symptoms of a "trapped nerve" when we talked about displaced pain and pins and needles. Displaced symptoms may come on suddenly after a fall or strained movement, or appear gradually, with no apparent cause. Sometimes injured ligaments can cause pain and numbness.

Gradual presentation of the symptoms usually means that the injury occurred earlier, often a day or two before. With such a chronic injury, something finally "gives" after struggling to cope for a long time. This is why the immediate cause of the pain is often some routine, apparently innocuous action.

A trapped nerve will cause displaced pain, and possibly also pins and needles or numbness. The pain is the nerve's way of letting you know it is distressed. The other symptoms of **altered sensation** are due to sensation not being transmitted normally by the distressed nerve.

There are several structures that can "trap" nerves. Nerves leave the spine through small gaps between the spinal bones or vertebrae. These gaps can be reduced in size by the restricted motion and muscle spasm of joint dysfunction, the growth of additional bone (called an osteophyte), or a spinal disc bulging. From the spine, the nerves then travel between the muscles of the neck. Nerves supplying the shoulder and arm also have to cross over the upper ribs. Dysfunction or damage in these areas can irritate the nerves.

Initial treatment is the same as for a neck sprain. Seek professional advice to determine exactly where the trouble is and how to treat it. Care is likely to involve manual treatment, exercise, and possibly electrotherapy. Conditions in which the nerve is severely impaired, or where other treatment fails, may need injections to block nerve function or require surgery to decompress the nerve.

If your symptoms are the result of a chronic problem, simply relieving the current irritation will not be enough. You need to address the long-term stresses that have built up. Work with a practitioner to reduce your overall patterns of mechanical stress and get help from a coach to correct any poor sporting technique. Adopting one of the postural therapies (see p.132) will often reap substantial rewards, too.

Thoracic outlet syndrome

This is a continuation of the trapped nerve idea. Here, both nerves and blood vessels that supply the arm are trapped. The pins and needles or numbness may be caused either by pressure on a nerve or by reduced blood flow through the arm. Pressure that impedes blood draining from the arm can also cause the hand to swell.

The pressure may occur in the side of the neck, between the collar bone and the top of the rib cage, or between the rib cage and chest muscles. Practitioners may check the pulse in your wrist, while you move your neck and arm. Finding the position that increases the pressure will cause your pulse to weaken or disappear.

Icing the neck is less useful here, particularly if the problem is further out in your shoulder. However, the condition is not usually an acute presentation, but is more typically a chronic buildup, so early diagnosis and treatment is the best option. Treatment targets the appropriate muscle and joints to restore normal movement. Improving the way you use your body is also important, particularly correcting slumped shoulder postures.

shoulder
injuries

We tend to think of shoulder movement as being the upper arm bone, or humerus, moving within the socket of the shoulder blade, but much more than that is involved.

The shoulder blade, or scapula, has to move to allow normal shoulder movement, and this requires movement at the joints between the shoulder blade and the collarbone, and the collarbone and the breastbone. The shoulder blade also has to glide smoothly over the back of the rib cage. Because the shoulder is connected to the head, neck, back, chest, pelvis, and arm, all these muscles influence it's movement.

Shoulder injuries are good examples of how dysfunction in one part of the body can cause symptoms elsewhere. For example, a soccer player who complained of pain and restricted movement in his right shoulder was found to have a strain in the joints of his pelvis. This influenced his shoulder through the latissimus dorsi, the large back muscle that links the pelvis and lower back to the arm.

Most shoulder problems have several components, with one dysfunction having a knock-on effect on others. While injuries are identified by the muscle or joint most directly involved, be prepared to look further afield for solutions.

Shoulder injuries are prevalent with throwing actions such as tennis and baseball pitching. Injuries also occur from falls onto the shoulder or outstretched arm.

Fractures and dislocations

Any of the bones or joints of the shoulder girdle can be fractured or dislocated. The commonest causes are falls and collisions.

The **collarbone** is the most frequently fractured bone in the body. Indications of damage are pain and swelling, with a change in the normal line of the bone (when compared with the other side).

Dislocations of the shoulder joint itself usually result in a "square shoulder," with a loss of the normal roundness of the side of the shoulder. Dislocations can be accompanied by fractures, so they should always be x-rayed before treatment.

Dislocation between the collarbone and shoulder blade can cause a visible bump on the top of the shoulder, as the end of the collarbone sticks up.

Less commonly, the inner end of the collarbone may dislocate from the breastbone. This requires emergency treatment if the collarbone moves backward, as it can press on the blood vessels to the head and arm.

Careful investigation and treatment of all fractures and dislocations is particularly important in the shoulder, as nerves and blood vessels supplying the arm can also be affected. In all cases, use a sling to limit movement and pain, and go to the hospital.

Injuries of muscles and tendons

Pain in the shoulder can originate in muscles in the neck, chest, or the shoulder itself. While the shoulder is a ball and socket joint, the socket on the shoulder blade is

Each of the players in this picture could have sustained a shoulder injury from this impact.

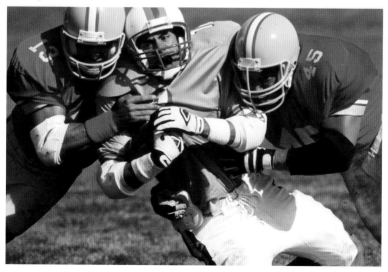

very shallow. This results in a joint that is extremely mobile, but not very stable. The **rotator cuff** muscles move the shoulder joint, but also aid shoulder stability by holding the ball of the arm bone into the socket of the shoulder blade.

Rotator cuff injuries These muscles and their tendons are involved in almost all shoulder actions. They can be damaged acutely as they attempt to stabilize the shoulder, such as when you put out your hand to save yourself in a fall. Chronically, they are prone to overuse injuries, particularly in racket sports, throwing activities, and swimming. Chronic injuries of the tendons are more likely from middle age onward.

The upper muscle of the group is the **supraspinatus**, which lies along a groove near the top of the shoulder blade. A tear of this muscle, or inflammation of its tendon, causes difficulty when you try to lift your arm up to the side.

To test this muscle, begin with your arm beside your body, then lift the arm up to the side, keeping your thumb pointing down to the ground, against resistance— either from your other arm, or preferably with somebody else pressing down for you. If pain occurs with this action, then it suggests a supraspinatus injury.

Swelling of the supraspinatus tendon causes "impingement," as the swollen part of the tendon is too wide to pass through its groove in the shoulder blade. This causes pain and prevents you lifting your arm out to the side fully.

The **infraspinatus** covers most of the back of the shoulder blade, and it acts to turn your arm outward. Test it by putting your hand out as if you were going to shake someone's hand, but keep your elbow by your side. Hold your hand in this position while your other hand tries to pull your wrist in across your body. If this produces pain, or is obviously weak, it indicates an infraspinatus injury.

The small **subscapularis** muscle is at the bottom of the shoulder blade and acts to turn your arm inward. It is a common site of injury. To test this muscle repeat the test above, but push your wrist sideways, away from the midline of your body.

If you have weakness in moving the shoulder, it is necessary to see a practitioner, as complete tears of the rotator cuff muscles or tendons may require surgical repair. Less severe injuries are treated initially by rest from activities that stress them, along with remedies to reduce inflammation. As the symptoms subside, begin a careful program of exercises to stretch and strengthen the shoulder muscles (see p.101).

PECTORALIS MUSCLE TEARS

The pectoralis major is the largest muscle of the chest. Extreme loading, such as heavy bench pressing, can cause tearing of this muscle. Minor tears are treated conservatively with RICE (Rest-Ice-Compression-Elevation) and progressive rehabilitation. Complete ruptures, however, are a surgical emergency. Symptoms include sudden severe pain over the front of the upper arm, just below the shoulder. This is followed by swelling and bruising over the same area, and weakness when trying to press the arm in toward the side of the body. Sometimes the shape of the muscle is visibly changed. If in any doubt, go directly to the hospital.

Trigger points Trigger points are tender nodules, usually found in muscles, that cause symptoms to be displaced to other parts of the body. A skilled manual therapist can locate trigger points, but, once found, you can often provide some of the treatment yourself. A simple method is to massage the area containing the trigger point with an ice cube, then gently stretch the muscle(s) containing the trigger point. Ask your practitioner for guidance. Shoulder and upper arm pain can be displaced from trigger points in the neck, upper chest, or the shoulder itself.

Subacromial bursitis This bursa provides cushioning between the shoulder joint and deltoid muscle. It can become inflamed by a fall, or chronic overstressing. Pain at the front of the shoulder is increased by lifting the arm to the side. The bursa lies over the supraspinatus tendon and can get trapped, causing impingement. You may feel a spongy, golf ball–size swelling on the outside of the shoulder. Acute cases are treated with RICE and anti-inflammatory remedies. Rare chronic cases require diagnosis of the mechanical problems. The bursa may be injected to relieve symptoms or removed surgically. This should only be considered if nonsurgical treatment has failed.

Systemic conditions Pain in the shoulder can be displaced from irritation of internal organs. If your pain is not significantly affected by movement, is present in all positions of rest, or is accompanied by fever, abdominal pain, jaundice, or unexplained weight loss, see your doctor for a diagnosis.

arm
and elbow
injuries

The elbow is a hinge joint, with movement being restricted to bending (flexion) and straightening (extension). The ability to turn the hand, which is essential for so many activities, requires movement between the two bones of the forearm. Slight restriction of this movement is a fairly common and often missed cause of elbow or wrist pain.

Most fractures heal with simple immobilization in a cast. Surgery may be needed for more complicated fractures, or where circulation or nerve conduction are affected.

Elbow dislocations are rare. When they do occur, they are often the result of a fall onto the hand when the elbow is bent. Signs of a dislocation are severe pain, swelling, and deformity of the elbow. Diagnosis is confirmed by an X-ray, which will also show up any associated fractures. Treatment involves relocating the bones to their appropriate positions, then splinting the elbow for seven to ten days. This should be followed by a programme of rehabilitation exercises.

FRACTURES AND DISLOCATIONS

Indications of a fracture include a traumatic injury causing pain and swelling, with possible deformation of the normal shape of the arm. Occasionally nerves and blood vessels lying near the bones are also damaged, so any examination should include checking circulation and sensation in the hand, as well as an X-ray.

Pain in the arm can be displaced from nerve irritation in the neck or from trigger points in the neck, chest, shoulder, or arm itself. As with all displaced pain, effective treatment requires identification of the source of the problem.

Loose bodies in the elbow

Elbow pain with stiffness and locking of the joint can be caused by small fragments of bone or cartilage floating loose in the elbow joint. This type of injury is most commonly caused by repeated throwing actions, such as is done by baseball pitchers. It is usually seen in adolescents, but can also occur in adults.

Symptoms may settle after rest from throwing, and manipulation of the elbow may help to resolve the problem. A progressive rehabilitation plan is then needed to build up strength and mobility in the area.

If symptoms do not subside, or if there is clear evidence of loose bodies on an X ray or scan, then surgery will be required, followed by rehabilitation.

Tennis and golfer's elbow

Tennis elbow is the most common cause of elbow pain. However, a significant number of patients diagnosed with "tennis elbow" become free of symptoms following treatment of their radial head dysfunction (see p.42), which suggests that this condition is sometimes misdiagnosed.

Tennis elbow is usually a strain of the tendon on the outer side of the elbow, which is the attachment point for several of the forearm muscles that extend (bend back) the wrist, as is used in tennis backhand. The name derives from its initial discovery in tennis players, where it was caused by excessive stress during such backhand strokes. The inner side of the elbow can also be affected by "golfer's elbow"—excessive strain on the wrist or forearm during tennis forehand or golfing swings. While it can be caused by a variety of sports, as well as gardening, tennis elbow is now very seldom seen in high-level tennis players. High-level players:

- Warm up effectively.
- Are well conditioned.
- Use a good technique.

This is often in distinct contrast to recreational players, in whom the problem is particularly common.

Signs of tennis elbow are pain on the outside of the elbow when you lift something with your palm pointing down. To test this, with your palm down, resist, as your other hand bends your wrist, by pushing the hand down toward the floor. If this reproduces the elbow pain, "tennis elbow" is likely.

Treatment requires rest from the causative actions, along with physical therapies to correct any underlying joint or muscle problems. Natural remedies and acupuncture can also speed up the healing process, as may photonic stimulation. A program of stretching and strengthening exercises will be needed to prevent reinjury.

Modify all causative factors. This means getting help to improve your technique and ensuring you are using suitable equipment, such as a racket that is not too tightly strung and has the right-sized grip.

A frequently used medical treatment is a steroid injection into the site of the injury, but this does not help all sufferers. If the injection fails, it may be that the patient was not accurately diagnosed, or the injection site was not precisely located. If all other treatment methods fail, surgery may be the solution.

Some people find benefit in "tennis elbow braces," which wrap around the forearm just below the elbow, and wrist splints. Their pressure limits the contraction of forearm muscles, thus reducing the pull on the tendon.

"Golfer's elbow" is the equivalent injury affecting the tendon on the inside of the elbow, and treatment is the same as for tennis elbow.

Radial head dysfunction

As already mentioned, the two bones of the forearm, the radius and ulna, need mobility in order to let your hand turn, such as when you need to turn a key in a lock. The two bones connect at the wrist and just below the elbow, which is where most of the movement takes place.

Restriction of movement can cause pain that is very close to the site of tennis elbow pain, and similar actions can aggravate the pain. This condition is thus often mistaken for tennis elbow. An osteopath or chiropractor should be able to palpate the movement, identify restrictions, and then manipulate the joint to restore movement.

Radial head dysfunction may cause pain in the wrist rather than the elbow. Again, skilled palpation is required to identify the real problem.

You can assist treatment with the following simple exercise. Clench the fist of the affected arm. Grip the wrist using your other hand, and maintain firm pressure. Circle your fist slowly in as big a circle as possible—go five times both clockwise and counterclockwise. If you keep your grip firm, the circles will be very small. Make sure that you take around three or four seconds to make each circle.

Muscle injuries

Minor strains to arm muscles occur in a wide range of sports, resulting in short-term localized pain. Treat these injuries with RICE (see p.104) and remedies to speed healing. Once the pain subsides, you should then begin a rehabilitation program (see p.138, and also ask your practitioner for guidance).

Biceps tendon injury

The long tendon of the biceps muscle runs through a bony groove at the top of the upper arm. The tendon can become inflamed at this point, can slip out of the groove completely, or can rupture. These problems are more likely if you have poor posture—if your shoulders are slumped or hunched forward.

Symptoms include pain in the front of the shoulder, which is increased by actions that involve bending the elbow, and turning the forearm palm upward against resistance. This often gives the impression of a shoulder problem rather than one located in the arm. A creaking feeling can sometimes be felt as the inflamed tendon rubs over the groove. A snapping sensation may also be felt if the tendon slips out of the groove.

Rupture of the tendon produces pain, swelling, and bruising at the front of the shoulder. You may be able to see the biceps muscle bunched up on the front of the arm.

Treatment of inflammation of the tendon (biceps tendonitis) is initially rest, application of ice, and anti-inflammatory remedies. You then need to check for dysfunction in the neck, upper back, and ribs, or muscular imbalance around the shoulder, to find the underlying cause of the problem. This will require the assistance of a manual and/or postural therapist.

If the tendon slips out of its groove, the condition may settle with conservative care, or may require surgical repair of the ligament that retains the tendon in the groove.

Rupture of the tendon requires emergency surgical repair. Delay in treatment will rapidly reduce the chances of success.

wrist
and hand
injuries

The hands are used in such a wide variety of sports that injuries affecting the wrist and hand are extremely common, and account for one quarter of all sporting injuries.

Skilled hand use, whether it is shooting a basket, catching a pass, or smashing a forehand, requires the hand to be in the right place and at the right angle. Hand function is dependent on arm function, and dysfunction of any part of the arm can cause wrist and hand injury.

The hands are the final point of expression for many sporting actions, putting them under considerable load.

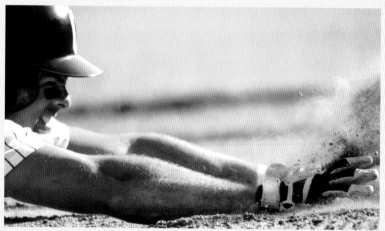

Poor hand positioning, due to restrictions in the shoulder or elbow, can strain the wrist and hand. Think of hand and wrist movements as the fine tuning elements of any sporting action. Movement and power production begin with foot positioning and body posture, before being transmitted through the arm, and finally expressed through the hand.

While considering the tissues involved in specific injuries of the wrist and hand, remember that wrist and hand symptoms can also be displaced from problems in the neck, shoulder, and arm.

Fractures and dislocations

Wrist fractures are commonly caused by a fall onto the outstretched hand or while tackling in rugby or football. Fractures of the radius and ulna (the bones of the forearm) cause pain, swelling, and often a deformity. These injuries are readily identified by X ray. Treatment requires correction of any malpositioning of the bones, followed by immobilization with a cast.

Fractures can also involve the carpals, the small bones of the wrist. The most frequently fractured of these is the scaphoid, which is found on the side of the wrist, under the base of the thumb.

Spread your thumb sideways away from the rest of your hand. Running from the back of the thumb down to the wrist you should be able to see two tendons. The hollow between these two tendons, where the wrist meets the hand, is known as the anatomical snuff box, and this is where the scaphoid lies.

It is important to know this because fractures of the scaphoid are often misdiagnosed as wrist sprains, and the resulting inappropriate treatment can cause long-term consequences. Scaphoid fractures are often not so dramatic, produce no visible deformity, and frequently do not show up on an initial X ray. Any "wrist sprain" with pain on the thumb side of the wrist, which does not resolve itself, should have a second X ray two weeks after the injury.

Scaphoid fractures require an extensive cast, from the middle of the upper arm to partway down the thumb. At least partial immobilization is often required for three to six months. Lack of treatment can cause part of the scaphoid to deteriorate due to a lack of blood supply, thus preventing healing. Fractures of hand or finger bones are usually the result of trauma in sports such as martial arts, basketball, and baseball. Signs are pain, swelling, and redness; fractured fingers may also be misshapen, sometimes looking twisted.

Treatment involves casting for a hand fracture, with surgical stabilization being needed for some injuries, particularly if the fracture involves a joint or the bone at the base of the thumb. Finger fractures may be splinted by a padded aluminium strip, which is anchored to a cast at the wrist.

Ligament injuries

Sprains to the wrist occur in gymnastics, where the hands carry body weight, and as a result of falls or collisions. Finger sprains are common from collisions where the finger is "knocked back." The most common hand injury of all is a sprain of the thumb.

Sprains vary in severity, depending on how many of the ligament fibers are torn. The symptoms of pain and swelling are likely to be greater the more severe the injury. A feeling of weakness in the joint is common, but a joint that is lax, i.e., that can move further than its normal range, suggests a more severe injury.

Initial treatment for all strains is RICE (see p.104). If the injury is not too severe, maintain mobility by keeping the joint moving within the **pain-free range**.

Moderately severe strains should be examined by a manual therapist, who will assess function in the joints around the injured joint. A fall onto the outstretched hand could cause problems in the hand, wrist, elbow, shoulder, neck, or upper back.

Severe strains producing laxity in a joint should be seen quickly by an orthopaedic surgeon, as surgical repair may be needed. More serious problems may include partial dislocation of one of the small bones in the wrist or the degeneration of the cartilage that supports the wrist.

Tendon injuries

Many of the muscles that move the wrist and hand are in the forearm, so tendons that connect the muscles to bones have to be long, and some have to get around several corners to allow complex hand movements. As a result, there are few muscle injuries, but more tendon injuries. Tendons exposed to high levels of stress or pressure are often protected by a sheath. Excessive levels of stress lead to inflammation of the sheath, or **tenosynovitis**. Like ligaments, tendons can be torn, the damage ranging from a few fibers to a complete rupture.

Mallet finger An impact, often from a ball, can bend the last joint of a finger forcefully, rupturing the tendon that pulls the finger straight. This results in one's being unable to straighten the finger normally, but one being able to straighten the finger with the other hand. Occasionally, the tendon pulls a small piece of bone away, so an X ray may be useful.

Treatment is in the form of a simple support that fits over the end of the finger, which holds the affected joint into a slightly backward bent position. This brings the torn ends of the tendon together and allows healing to take place, which is usually complete after about six weeks.

Jersey finger This is a rupture of the tendon that bends the last joint of a finger. If the pull is strong enough to tear the tendon, the person has difficulty bending the joint. Bruising is often visible on the palm side of the finger.

These injuries require prompt professional treatment, as the tendon can be pulled into the hand by muscle contraction. This condition necessitates early surgical repair.

Tenosynovitis Inflammation of a tendon (tendonitis) or its sheath (tenosynovitis) are injuries resulting from overuse, occurring in sports that place high loads on the wrist and hand, such as racket sports, gymnastics, and rowing. This can include the extended use of rowing machines in health clubs or the home.

Symptoms are pain with particular movements, a creaking sensation over the tendon with movement, and tenderness. Which movements produce pain and creaking will depend on which tendon is affected. The most common site of damage is around the wrist near the thumb.

Prevention is the best treatment, which, as usual, involves thorough warming up, progressive training, and the use of good technique and appropriate equipment at all times. Once injured, a tendon will need rest, as continued loading will cause chronic inflammation and the likelihood of fibrosis and adhesions, resulting in a permanent problem.

Rest may be accompanied by anti-inflammatory remedies. The correction of any underlying muscle or joint dysfunction is vital for long-term prevention, and in persistent cases steroid injections provide effective relief from symptoms (see p. 106).

back
injuries

Back problems in general are extremely common, and are the result of many factors including poor posture, misuse, repetitive injuries, and inadequate ergonomics. In many instances where back problems appear to be sporting injuries, sport was not the real cause – it was just the final straw on an already overloaded camel.

The back is severely loaded in weight lifting and rowing, and exposed to repeated loading, particularly linked with rapid and extreme movements, in gymnastics, figure skating, diving, tennis, and golf.

Preventing back problems

More than any other area, prevention of back injuries goes beyond considering your sporting activity. Consider all aspects of your life, including general posture, work ergonomics, and leisure activities, to prevent the overall load on your back from building to a point where something has to give.

Good physical conditioning for the back, which is an integral part of sports conditioning, helps prevent not just sport-related injury, but also general back problems. This is an example of how well-managed sporting activity contributes to your overall well-being. Good functioning of the back, like any other part of the body, requires a balance of stability and flexibility. Distorted postures are often the result of poor control patterns. Most of us, usually as teenagers, have been told to "stand up straight". However, with no internal blueprint for what "stand up straight" means, our heroic physical efforts just produce an even more distorted and rigid posture. These postures waste huge amounts of energy and are impossible to sustain. As soon as you attend to anything else, habit takes over and you slump back to your old familiar pose.

Changing how you use your body requires a method for raising awareness of what you are doing now, and tools to make practical change. The resulting increase in freedom and grace, and the decrease in wear and tear, is well worth the investment required. The section on postural therapies beginning on p.132 introduces some of the effective methods that are available.

Signs of back injuries

Pain from a back injury can range from the stiff, achy feeling you might get a day or two after unaccustomed exercise to severe pain that leaves you bedridden. A key identifier of pain caused by a mechanical injury is that it will be affected by movement or posture.

Pain due to spinal joint sprains in the upper back will often be irritated by deep breathing movements or turning to look over your shoulder. Lower back pains are likely to be influenced by sitting, standing, bending, or walking.

Back injury can also displace pain around the ribs to the chest, into the groin, or down into the buttocks or legs. Where pain is displaced to depends on where

---

Sports involving extreme positions can expose the back to an increased risk of injury.

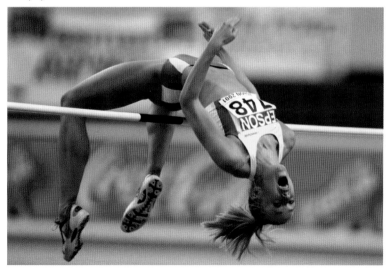

in the back the injury is; its origins may be in the joints of the vertebrae, in muscles, or from compromised ligaments. Injuries that put pressure on nerves coming from the spine can also cause pins and needles or numbness.

Pain that is unaffected by position or movement may be displaced to the back from internal organs. Certain characteristics of back pain require a full medical evaluation, as they are unlikely to be produced by a sports injury.

- **Unremitting pain**—Pain that is constant and is not altered by rest, position, or movement. Pain that is deep and penetrating in quality.
- **Systemic signs**—Pain that is associated with signs of general ill health, including fever, unexplained weight loss, night sweats, enlarged lymph nodes, or alteration in bowel or bladder habit. (Some pain-killing medications used for back pain can cause constipation. If in doubt about any medications you are using, consult your doctor or pharmacist.)

Muscle spasm

This can occur as a result of a sudden movement, an excessive load, or an impact leading to a muscle strain. Pain will be localized to the injured muscle, increased

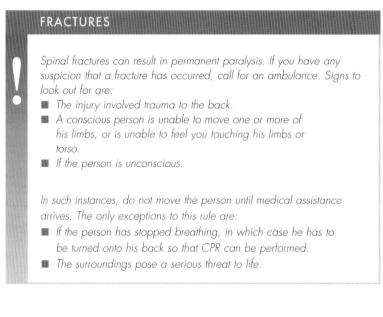

FRACTURES

Spinal fractures can result in permanent paralysis. If you have any suspicion that a fracture has occurred, call for an ambulance. Signs to look out for are:

- *The injury involved trauma to the back.*
- *A conscious person is unable to move one or more of his limbs, or is unable to feel you touching his limbs or torso.*
- *If the person is unconscious.*

In such instances, do not move the person until medical assistance arrives. The only exceptions to this rule are:

- *If the person has stopped breathing, in which case he has to be turned onto his back so that CPR can be performed.*
- *The surroundings pose a serious threat to life.*

by activities that stretch or load the muscle, and relieved by positions that relax the muscle. Bruising may appear with injury to superficial muscles.

Rest and the application of ice should bring improvement within a few days, but the time taken for full healing will depend on the severity of the injury. Once healing is well under way, stretching and strengthening is important to prevent recurrence.

Persistent muscle spasm suggests an underlying problem, usually a **joint dysfunction** or a **trigger point**.

Joint injuries

There are a variety of structures within the back that can be injured, including joints, discs, muscles, and ligaments, which makes the diagnosis of back injuries often very complex. Back pain is frequently diagnosed as "muscular" if there is back pain alone, or a "slipped disc" if pain radiates into the leg. The former vague diagnosis often produces no effective treatment; the latter frightens the sufferer into inactivity.

Spinal joint dysfunction Joint dysfunction describes a situation in which there is a restriction of normal movement at a joint, with associated muscle spasm, and often with tenderness and pain. Dysfunction may be the result of severe acute strain, or long-term microstrains resulting from poor posture or repeated movements. Pain is usually aggravated by one or more movements, depending on which joint movements are restricted.

Pain from joint dysfunction in the upper back is often displaced outward from the spine, so that it is felt under the shoulder blade. It may be aggravated by movements of the back, head, or arms, such as deep breathing or coughing. The joints where the ribs connect to the spine can also be strained, with the possibility of pain being displaced around to the chest.

Joint dysfunction in the lower back may be displaced to the groin, hip, buttock, or leg, and may be aggravated or relieved by sitting, bending, twisting, or lying. Pain displaced down the leg that is made worse by coughing or straining bowel movements may be caused by a disc problem.

Initial care involves rest from irritating activities, the application of ice, and anti-inflammatory remedies. Treatment of joint dysfunction requires manipulation to reduce muscle spasm and restore normal joint movement.

The spine functions as a unit and should be treated as a whole. Restoring spinal function may require treatment of distant areas that influence the function of the spine, including muscles, ligaments, and joints anywhere in the body from the jaw to the feet. Osteopaths and chiropractors tend to look at problems in this way, seeing them within the context of the person as a whole.

Sacroiliac joint sprain The sacroiliac joints connect the bones at the back of the pelvis. They lie one to two inches out from the midline, at the top of the buttocks. Unlike shoulders or knees, these joints do not have big obvious movements, but their movements are still important. They allow a degree of "give" in the pelvis, preventing the damage that would occur otherwise due to the large forces that pass through the pelvis when we run or jump.

Sacroiliac sprains are caused by movements that place imbalanced stresses on the pelvis, such as falling onto one buttock or extreme lunging movements onto one leg. They are also often the result of relatively minor, but unguarded movements, such as stepping off a curb unexpectedly.

Pain is likely in the buttock, but can also radiate into the hip, groin, and down the back of the thigh as far as the knee or even the foot. Movements that stress the joint will influence the pain, such as bending forward or backward, sitting down or standing up, and walking. How movements or positions affect the pain will depend on which way the joint has been sprained. Treatment requires manipulation to reduce muscle spasm and restore normal movement. If lax ligaments are to blame, prolotherapy can be effective (see p.137).

"Slipped disc" Contrary to popular belief, discs do not "slip," and disc problems are not common. Intervertebral discs are made of cartilage, with a fibrous outer **casing** and a gel-like filling. They absorb shock and allow movement between adjacent vertebrae in the spine.

With long-term abuse, the outer fibers can suffer many small tears, until eventually the wall of the disc bulges outward under pressure from the gel inside. The bulge can press on the nerve leaving the spine, causing pain, pins and needles, numbness, and weakness in the skin and muscles supplied by the nerve. Occasionally, the onset is rapid after a traumatic injury. More commonly, symptoms come on insidiously, with no obvious trigger, but following a history of episodic lower back pain. The pain is often severe, and more in the leg than the back. Pins and needles, tingling, or numbness occur in part of the leg and/or foot. The sufferer is often unable to stand up straight, but this in itself does not confirm the diagnosis of a disc injury.

Treatment is initially rest and application of ice, plus anti-inflammatory remedies or pain relieving medications. Oral or injected steroids are reserved for severe symptoms, such as loss of sensation in the lower limbs (see p.106).

The pain may force bed rest but this should be limited to two or three days. Lie in whatever is the most comfortable posture—let pain be your guide.

Even though the worst pain may be in the leg, you should apply ice packs to your lower back, where the pain is coming from. Ensure that you have some thin material between the ice pack and your skin in order to prevent ice burns. Apply this for 20 minutes every two hours.

Most disc problems will settle with conservative care from a manual therapist. Occasionally, surgery is required to remove the bulging part of the disc. See a surgeon quickly if numbness or weakness continues to increase after the initial onset, or if control of your bowels or bladder is affected.

Sciatica This is pain radiating down the back of the leg, sometimes even as far as the foot. Sciatica, like a headache, is a symptom not a diagnosis. There are a number of mechanisms that can produce sciatica, and effective treatment requires identification of the cause. Possibilities include the sprain of lumbar spinal or sacroiliac joints or ligaments, a trigger point in the buttock, or a disc problem.

Trigger points are taut bands or knots in muscles that are felt as "tense" hard nodules. They are a very common cause of back pain and, as they create symptoms distant from themselves, they are often missed. Trigger points in the back, neck, shoulder, or abdomen can all lead to back pain. Causes of trigger points include acute or repetitive strains, or spinal joint sprains.

Treatment requires deactivation of the trigger point, followed by stretching to restore normal length to the muscle. See manual therapies beginning on p.108 for further information.

chest
injuries

While not the commonest of sports injuries, there are several chest injuries worth being aware of. The most frequently presenting problems are contusions or fractures from collisions, and muscle strains.

Fractures

Potential injury sites are the ribs, collar bones, and the breast bone. Collar bone fractures are covered in shoulder injuries on p.36, while breast bone fractures are extremely rare in the context of sports injuries.

The usual uncomplicated rib fractures are treated with rest and pain relief, which may consist of pharmaceutical or natural remedies. Strapping or taping tends to limit breathing movement and lung function, so it is not normally used. Often X-rays are not taken as treatment will be the same whether you have fractured a rib or not.

! **FRACTURES**

Rib fractures are usually the result of trauma to the chest, as in tackles or impact from a hard ball or puck. They produce pain, tenderness, and sometimes swelling over the injury site. Pain is aggravated by deep breathing, coughing, or pressure anywhere on the chest.

Even shallow breathing may be painful but, if breathlessness develops, you should get to a hospital quickly, as the broken end of a rib can damage the lung.

Rarely, in a severe impact, several ribs on both sides of the chest may be fractured, leaving the chest wall relatively unstable. This "flail chest" injury requires hospital investigation.

Joint sprains

Chest pain can result from sprains of any of the joints within the "thoracic cage," or bony part of the chest. Each rib consists of a bony part and a cartilage part. The joint between the two parts can be sprained, as can the joints between the breast bone and ribs or the ribs and the spine. Joint sprains can occur with impacts to the chest or upper back, but equally they can be caused by strenuous movements, particularly those involving twisting or bending sideways.

Pain is made worse with deep breathing or movements that challenge the sprained joint. The presentation is similar to that for a rib fracture, and differentiating between the two can be difficult. Initial treatment is rest and application of ice, with anti-inflammatory remedies. A manual therapist will help to restore normal movement to the joint and reduce any associated muscle spasm. Acupuncture may also be useful to reduce inflammation and spasm by restoring normal energy flow.

Muscle strain

The large pectoral muscles of the chest are used in actions such as pushing forward and any movements involving drawing the upper arm toward the chest. It is during these actions, with excessive effort, that pectoral muscle strains are likely. See shoulder injuries on p.39 for information on pectoral muscle rupture.

Localized pain and tenderness, possibly with bruising, are symptoms. Stretching the muscle, or contracting it against resistance, will increase the pain.

Rest and application of ice are the first measures, along with anti-inflammatory remedies and/or acupuncture. Once healing is underway, rehabilitation requires progressive exercise to strengthen and stretch the muscle within pain-free limits.

Breast and nipple injuries

A common problem is "jogger's nipple"—soreness and inflammation caused by repeated friction between clothing and a nipple. The simple remedy is either to stick an adhesive dressing over the nipple to act as a shield or to put a blob of petroleum jelly over the nipple to act as a lubricant.

Bras should be well-fitting for sporting activity, as excessive breast movement frequently causes pain for women involved in activities such as running or high-impact aerobics. A well-fitting sports bra is most effective at reducing this discomfort.

hip
and groin
injuries

This area contains the biggest muscles in the body, and the ones most responsible for moving us around. As much of sporting activity is simply "moving us around" taken towards its limit, you can see why injuries, particularly muscle strains, are very common.

Hip joint injuries

Fractures and dislocations are rare sporting injuries in adults. Fractures of the pelvis can occur with forceful impacts such as motor sport crashes. Hip pain or prolonged limping in a child requires investigation.

Joint dysfunction

Pain in the hip area can result from the dysfunction of lower back joints, the sacro iliac joints at the back of the pelvis, the symphysis pubis at the front of the pelvis, the joint with the coccyx or tail bone, and the hip joint itself. Lower back and sacro iliac joints are covered in back injuries, starting on p.48.

Symphysis pubis The symphysis pubis is the joint at the front of the pelvis in the groin. It can be sprained by heavy or repeated uneven loading, like landing on one leg when jumping down from a height. Extra care is needed during pregnancy, when the pelvic joints soften for childbirth.

Pain occurs in the lower back, buttock, groin, or even as far down as the inner side of the knee. Standing on one leg may increase the pain. Manual therapy is used to restore normal joint function.

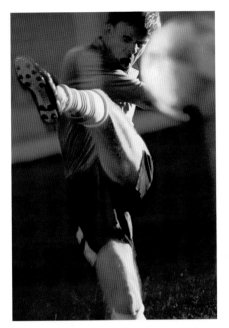

The hip joint is acted upon by the largest muscles in the body.

Hip joint Dysfunction of the hip joint is often due to muscle imbalance caused by training or sports that overemphasize the development of some muscles at the expense of others. Hip dysfunction is likely to present itself as pain or repeated injury of muscles that are struggling to cope with the imbalance—recurrent "groin strains," for example. A manual therapist can diagnose and correct joint dysfunction and underlying muscle imbalance. These are addressed with exercises to stretch tight, and strengthen weak, muscles. Postural therapies, such as the Alexander technique, can help you to recognize and address habits in the way you use yourself, which cause muscle imbalance around the hips and pelvis. Many systems that focus on body use place great emphasis on the importance of pelvic posture.

Coccyx dysfunction The joint between the pelvis and the coccyx (or tail bone) can be injured by a direct blow. Pain, which can be extreme, is felt between the buttocks, and is often made worse by sitting. A doughnut-shaped cushion is often helpful. Treatment is rest and application of ice, followed by manipulative therapy to restore normal function and position of the coccyx. An X ray may identify a fracture. Pain-relieving and steroid injections are often prescribed in severe cases.

Contusions

A fall, or collision with another player, causes pelvic contusions. Expect pain, tenderness, and often bruising at the injury site. Sliding along the ground, particularly on synthetic surfaces, causes skin abrasions. Bleeding often occurs in the large pelvic muscles or in the abdominal muscles where they attach to the top of the pelvis. This results in a **haematoma,** or pool of blood, within the tissues. Similar injuries affect the abdominal muscles as a result of bending the body forcefully sideways—when receiving a tackle, for example.

As with all muscle strains, apply RICE (see p.104). If the skin is damaged, it should be cleaned and dressed to prevent infection. Avoid NSAIDs, as these can increase the bleeding. For the same reason, don't apply heat or massage initially.

As symptoms settle, start stretching exercises to restore normal movement, followed by strengthening exercises. A manual therapist can assist you.

Muscle injuries

These are the most frequent injuries affecting this area, and include tightness produced by spasm and the varying degrees of tearing or strain. Causes and symptoms vary depending on the muscle affected, so they are detailed individually. However, muscles are unlikely to be injured without other parts of the body being involved. The exercise section beginning on p.97 explains how to stretch specific muscles.

Adductor muscles The hip adductor muscles run down the inside of the thigh and bring the legs together. They are strained by overstretching or by a strong contraction when changing direction to one side. This is the classic "groin strain," with pain in the groin or inner thigh area that limits hip movements, possibly with bruising. Treat with RICE initially, followed by manual therapy to reduce muscle spasm and improve circulation. Natural remedies can also help accelerate the healing process.

Complete rupture of a muscle, with bunching of the shortened muscle on the inner thigh, requires surgical repair. Reinjury is common. Prevent it by thorough rehabilitation to restore strength and increase flexibility. Adductor strain often results from tightness in the buttock muscles, so include exercises that stretch them.

Hip flexors The hip flexors allow you to bend at the hips and bring your knees in toward your torso. Injury often makes standing up straight painful or difficult. These muscles are widely used, and are often short due to prolonged sitting, making injuries more likely.

Strain can occur from any activity that lifts your leg up in front, including running. Pain can be felt in the groin, down the front of the thigh, or in the lower back. Treatment is the same as for adductor strain. The strongest hip flexor attaches to the lumbar spine, so treatment may need to include attention to lumbar spinal joints.

Piriformis This muscle lies deep in your buttock. It is the main muscle for turning your leg outward, and is often tight. If you tend to stand with your feet pointing out at "ten to two," both sides are probably tight. Piriformis spasm causes buttock pain or pain down the back of the leg mimicking sciatica. Turning your leg inward, which stretches the piriformis, will aggravate the symptoms. Treatment must address any underlying problem, along with exercises to stretch the piriformis.

Quadratus lumborum Quadratus lumborum spasm is a common cause of lower back pain, but trigger points in these muscles displace pain to the buttock or down the side of the hip. Hip pain with no local cause, which is made worse if you bend to the opposite side, may be caused by a quadratus lumborum trigger point. Treatment involves deactivation of the trigger point, followed by muscle stretching.

Bursitis

Trochanteric bursitis The greater trochanter is the bony lump at the top of the outside of your thigh. Tenderness and swelling just below the trochanter, with pain that is sent down the outside of the thigh, suggests trochanteric bursitis (an inflammation of the "front cushions"), which may cause swelling. Symptoms are usually aggravated by walking or lifting the leg out sideways.

Treat with rest, application of ice, and anti-inflammatory remedies, or, in severe cases, pain-relieving or steroid injections (see p.106), then check for underlying mechanical strains around the hip. If symptoms follow a blow to the hip, suspect bleeding into the bursa, which may require medical draining with a syringe.

Psoas bursitis Inflammation of this bursa causes pain and swelling in the groin, irritated by lifting the knee against resistance. This condition can be confused with a hip muscle or tendon problem. It can also cause a "clicky hip." Treatment is the same as for trochanteric bursitis, but, in extreme cases, surgery may be required.

thigh
injuries

Thigh injuries occur frequently and most of them are muscular, with hamstring strains being the most common.

Contusions

Blows to the upper leg are a common occurrence in many contact sports, including soccer and rugby. The quadriceps muscles on the front of the thigh are the most frequently affected – this is sometimes known as "Charley horse" injury.

The onset of a contusion is usually obvious, with pain and later bruising. Bleeding into the muscle forms a haematoma, and poor management of this can result in **myositis ossificans**, where bone forms within the injury site. This can permanently restrict flexibility of the muscle and increase the risk of re-injury.

The aim of initial treatment is to limit the bleeding, which is achieved by applying RICE. *No heat or massage should be used at this stage.* Once the risk of bleeding is reduced, two to three days after the injury, gentle static isometric contractions of the quadriceps (tightening the quadriceps muscle at the front of the thigh) will stimulate circulation into the area. Returning to activity too early causes re-injury with more bleeding, and it is persistent bleeding that can lead to bone formation within the muscle. Ensure that progressive return to activity is pain free to prevent this.

FRACTURES

! *Fractures of the thigh bone or femur are extremely rare sporting injuries among adults. They are sometimes seen in children, often just above the knee. The onset would be due to a severe trauma, with swelling and extreme pain preventing movement. The bone must be realigned before casting.*

Muscle strains

Strains are caused by movements that stretch the muscle beyond its limits or by explosive movements where the muscle contracts forcefully, causing damage. They vary in severity from minor injuries, which resolve in two to three days, to complete ruptures needing surgical repair. Muscle strains are more likely with poor conditioning, insufficient warm-up, and poor technique.

Hamstrings A graphic example of a hamstring strain is the sprinter who pulls up limping and grabbing the back of his thigh after accelerating out of the blocks. The pain is sudden and stabbing in nature, and in a severe strain may be accompanied by a popping sensation in the back of the thigh. Attempting to bend forward with the knees straight or trying to bend the knee against resistance will increase the pain. The lump of a bunched-up muscle suggests a complete rupture, demanding the attention of an orthopaedic surgeon.

Treatment of incomplete tears is RICE, followed by progressive pain-free stretching and strengthening exercises as the symptoms begin to settle. Natural remedies can also be useful in resolving the bruising and helping to speed up healing.

Quadriceps Tears of the quadriceps at the front of the thigh occur with forceful actions such as jumping. Pain may be felt in the thigh or in the groin, where part of the muscle attaches to the pelvis. Swelling is greater the more severe the strain, and pain is increased by bending the knee. Treatment is the same as for hamstring strain.

Iliotibial band syndrome This condition is most common among runners. For more information see p.66.

Displaced pain Even when it is severe, displaced pain is often vague in its location. The painful area is not usually tender to the touch, and local treatment, such as massage, has a very limited impact.

Pain can be displaced to the thigh as a result of nerve irritation caused by lower back problems. If your pain goes below the knee, if you have pins and needles or numbness, or if your pain is influenced by moving your back, suspect a back problem (see p.48). Trigger points in the buttocks or within the thigh can also cause thigh pain.

knee
injuries

The knee is the largest joint in the body and the one most often troubled by sports injuries. Its job is to maintain stability with mobility, while being acted on by powerful muscles, through long levers, and at the same time support the body's weight. The fact that it manages so well is a testament to our miraculous human design.

Knees are injured acutely by direct trauma or by uncoordinated movements. Chronic injuries are caused by prolonged poor use, compromised function in other areas (such as the hip, foot, or ankle), and by severe overuse.

FRACTURES AND DISLOCATIONS

! *Fractures of the knee are relatively rare and are associated with extreme pain, swelling, and possible deformity of the joint.*

A less obvious problem is osteochondritis desicans, where a small fragment of cartilage and bone is broken off the thigh bone inside the knee joint. This problem occurs most in boys. Symptoms are vague pain, often mild swelling, and, in some cases, locking and giving way of the knee. Diagnosis is confirmed by an X-ray or arthroscopy, where a tiny fibre optic probe is inserted into the joint. Young sufferers often respond excellently to rest but adults may require surgery.

Knee dislocations are rare and usually easy to spot. Dislocations of the knee cap or patella happen more frequently. Usually the knee cap is displaced sideways, towards the outer side of the leg, and may pop back into place as the knee is straightened. Even if it does pop back, examination in a hospital is essential as soft tissues that hold the knee cap in place may be damaged.

Patello-femoral pain

As your knee bends and straightens, your kneecap, or **patella,** should glide smoothly up and down in the groove at the end of your thigh bone. Pain felt "behind the kneecap" is often caused by the kneecap rubbing on the thigh bone. In extreme cases, the smooth cartilage surface on the back of the kneecap begins to crack and break down, a condition known as **chondromalacia patella**.

Pain is worse when the knee is loaded in a bent position, such as during squatting actions or walking up or down hills or steps. Prolonged sitting in a cramped space, such as on a plane or in a theater, may cause aching in the knee.

The problem is often caused by an imbalance in the quadriceps muscles on the front of the thigh, which means the kneecap is pulled more toward the outside. Other causes include falls onto the knees and poor foot mechanics, sometimes due to faulty sports shoes.

Treatment requires reducing the impact from running or jumping, along with strengthening and stretching exercises for the quadriceps. A variety of straps or supports are available to improve the "tracking" of the kneecap, which can reduce symptoms until you find and treat the underlying cause.

Cartilage (meniscus) injuries

Within the knee, there are two crescent-shaped cartilages, or **menisci**. These improve the fit between the thighbone and shinbone, and act as shock absorbers. Cartilage tears are often the result of twisting strains while the knee is bent.

The **medial** cartilage on the inner side of the knee is injured much more frequently than the **lateral**

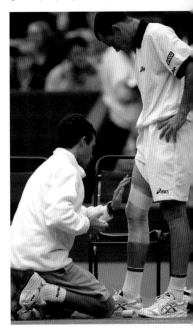

Appropriate strapping can support ligament injuries during their recovery.

cartilage. Pain occurs on the side of the knee where the cartilage is damaged, and other signs include swelling, "clicking," locking, and giving way of the knee.

Initial treatment is rest, application of ice, and exercises to maintain or increase the strength of the quadriceps muscles at the front of the thigh. If this settles the problem, begin a program of rehabilitation, checking the stability of your knee under progressively increasing loads, prior to a return to sporting activity.

If the symptoms do not fully resolve, an orthopaedic surgeon should perform an arthroscopy to examine the knee. Some cartilage tears can be surgically repaired. In other cases, the surgeon will perform a **partial menisectomy**, where the torn fragments are removed, leaving as much healthy cartilage intact as possible. Modern surgical techniques are followed by immediate rehabilitation exercises, often with a return to sports within a few weeks.

Injuries may involve cartilage alone, or may also be complicated by ligament damage.

Ligament injuries

Ligament ruptures damage knee stability drastically and often require surgery. With less severe sprains, increasing the stabilizing action of muscles can reduce the load on the ligaments, allowing the condition to settle down. As a rule of thumb in acute ligament injuries, the greater the amount of swelling the more serious the injury.

Medial collateral ligament This is the ligament that runs down the inner side of your knee, linking the thigh and shin bones. It can be sprained by forces pushing the foot out sideways or the knee inward and by twisting strains on a bent knee.

The medial collateral ligament is connected to the medial cartilage, so injuries are often associated with cartilage damage as well.

Pain on the inside of the knee is immediate, and may be followed by swelling and/or bruising of the area. The knee will often feel unstable, and any attempt at sporting activity should be stopped immediately.

Treat with RICE (see p.104) and, if the injury seems severe, arrange an early hospital examination in case surgery is required. For less severe problems, see a manual therapist as soon as possible. Mild sprains should be iced for 20 minutes two or three times a day, and a support bandage then used. Avoid stressing the ligament in this early stage, and limit the weight bearing down on it by using a crutch. Gentle mobility exercises are used to prevent stiffness.

After one to two weeks, strengthening exercises can be initiated, along with a return to normal weight bearing. After four weeks, the rehabilitation should be increased, working toward a return to sports when the knee is pain-free. The rehabilitation should progress so that you gain maximum improvement without damaging the repairing ligament. Ask your manual therapist if you would like help in managing this process.

Severe sprains require more prolonged rehabilitation. Complete tears, which are often associated with anterior cruciate ligament damage, may require surgical repair. The use of a hinged knee brace can allow for greater activity without overly stressing the repairing ligament.

Lateral collateral ligament This runs down the outer side of the knee, and is injured much less often than the medial collateral ligament. Strains occur when the knee is forced outward or if the foot is pushed inward.

Symptoms are the same as for medial collateral ligament, except that all the signs are on the outside of the knee. The lateral ligament does not suffer the added complication of connection to the lateral cartilage.

Treatment is as for medial collateral ligament; surgery is rarely needed.

Cruciate ligaments Right inside the knee joint itself are two ligaments forming a cross, hence the name **cruciate**. Together they help to stabilize the knee against forward and backward sliding motions. These ligaments may be injured acutely by severe stresses on the knee or may be injured chronically by repeated smaller stresses caused by a faulty technique in training or performance. Chronic injuries often present themselves as minor versions of acute injuries, which are detailed below.

Anterior cruciate ligament The anterior cruciate is injured more frequently than the posterior, usually by a very forceful twisting or side-bending action. The medial collateral ligament is often injured at the same time, leading to a very unstable knee.

Signs of this injury are instantaneous pain, sometimes accompanied by an audible "pop" if the ligament is ruptured completely; the knee gives way and swells very quickly. This swelling is due to bleeding from the torn ligament into the joint space. The pressure that this produces causes pain, which increases with the amount of swelling. A doctor can relieve this pressure by draining the blood using a syringe, known as **aspirating** the joint.

Anyone with this degree of injury should be transferred to a hospital for treatment as quickly as possible. If you can, use ice to help control the bleeding during the journey to the hospital.

Treatment is dependent on the severity of the injury. Partial tears are treated with exercises to strengthen the structures around the knee while the ligament is repairing. A hinged knee brace may be recommended to stabilize the joint during activity.

Complete tears may require surgical repair, depending on the degree of damage to, the age of, and the sporting expectations of the sufferer. Full rehabilitation can take up to a year.

Posterior cruciate ligament Injuries to this ligament occur as a result of falling onto a bent knee or the twisting of a straight knee. The back of the joint capsule is often torn at the same time, allowing blood to leak out of the joint capsule. Severe swelling and the associated pain is less likely than with an anterior cruciate tear. Tenderness at the back of the knee may also be present.

A medical examination is necessary to differentiate which tissues have been damaged, and to decide on the appropriate treatment.

Iliotibial band syndrome

A strong band of connective tissue known as the **iliotibial band,** or **fascia lata,** runs down the outside of your thigh. Many runners experience pain on the outside of their knees where this band rubs across the bone—a condition known as "runner's knee." Pain with a characteristic burning quality may also run down the outside of the thigh.

This pain can be caused by a tight iliotibial band due to excessive muscle tension in the hip, faulty foot mechanics, and poor choice of shoes. Treatment must deal with the cause, and so it may include manual therapy to correct lower limb mechanics, exercises to stretch tight muscles, obtaining "orthotic" inserts for your shoes from a podiatrist, or changing your running shoes.

Running on the same side of cambered roads or banked tracks can cause problems, as pelvic muscles are strained more on one side than the other.

Osgood-Schlatter disease

Strain where the tendon from the quadriceps muscles inserts into the top of the shinbone causes inflammation. It usually occurs in the 12–16 age group, affecting boys more than girls, and in the past it has been misdiagnosed as "growing pains." It is an overuse injury, causing pain with activity, and a tenderness on the shinbone just below the kneecap.

Treatment involves reducing activity to allow the condition to settle. Have a manual therapist check for any mechanical dysfunction causing increased stress on the area. There are no long-term consequences to this condition.

Jumper's knee

Also called **patella tendonitis**, this is a sprain of the quadriceps tendon, where it attaches to the top of the kneecap. It is caused by overloading with repeated forceful contractions of the quadriceps, such as in jumping.

There is intermittent swelling and pain when the quadriceps contract strongly. Initial treatment is rest and the application of ice, followed by ice massage to the area. Long-term correction requires exercises to stretch and strengthen the quadriceps and the resolution of any associated mechanical dysfunction by a manual therapist.

Bursitis

There are several bursae around the knee, and they can become inflamed as a result of direct trauma or by excessive stresses to surrounding tissues.

Symptoms are localized pain, swelling, heat, and tenderness. Treatment is with RICE initially (see p.104), and the reduction of any irritating stresses by resolving mechanical dysfunction and correcting training habits. Infected or chronically inflamed bursae are sometimes treated with steroid injections or with surgery.

lower leg
injuries

Trauma and muscular strains make up the bulk of injuries affecting the lower leg.

Stress fractures are overuse injuries, mostly seen in distance runners or from activities involving repeated jumping such as gymnastics. Causative factors include rapid increases in mileage, running on hard surfaces, and foot problems. Symptoms include localized pain and tenderness, the pain being worse with activity. An X-ray will provide a definitive diagnosis, although stress fractures can be difficult to spot.

Treatment involves stopping activities involving impact to the leg, and maintaining fitness with non-impact activities such as rowing. Ice massage can provide pain relief. Casting is not often required as the fracture is through part of the bone only.

FRACTURES

There are two bones in the lower leg: the tibia and the fibula. Fractures can affect them individually or together, and may be acute or chronic "stress" fractures.

Acute fractures will be traumatic in origin, cause severe pain and swelling and usually stop the victim from bearing weight on the leg. Fibular fractures may be less severe than tibial fractures, as the tibia is the main weight-bearing bone. Trauma may be obvious, such as a kick to the leg in soccer, or less obvious, such as the leg being forced against the top of a rigid ski boot during a fall.

Treatment is by immobilization with a cast. Complicated fractures may also require surgery to position and stabilize bone fragments with pins or wire.

Shinsplints

This is another overuse injury, often associated with increases in running mileage, hard running surfaces, or increases in training intensity. Pain and occasionally mild swelling occur on the inner edge of the tibia, or shinbone. The name shinsplints is gradually being replaced with the term **medial tibial stress syndrome**.

The symptoms are similar to a tibial stress fracture, but the pain and tenderness is more diffuse, often spreading over half the length of the shin. The pain is also aggravated either by moving the foot up or down against resistance. Rest from the causative activities is important, along with strengthening and stretching exercises to improve lower-leg muscle function. Stretching of the calf muscle and achilles tendon is particularly important. Hip, knee, or foot and ankle problems can be underlying causes, so have the function of these areas checked in order to prevent recurrence.

Contusions

Blows to the lower leg are common, particularly in soccer, and injuries can be very painful. It is important to rule out the possibility of a **fracture** or the onset of an

All running and kicking activities concentrate loads on the lower leg.

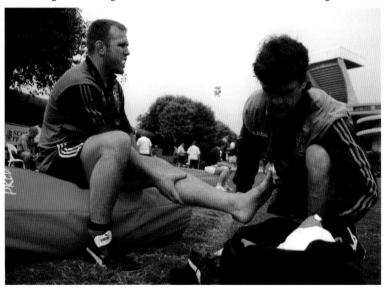

acute compartment syndrome. A blow to the outside of the lower leg can damage the **peronial nerve** leading to "foot drop," caused by muscle weakness.

Initially a fracture must be ruled out, and **fibular joint dysfunction** should also be checked for. A brace may be needed to hold the foot up to prevent tripping, but the condition usually resolves itself with time. Electrical stimulation can help exercise the muscles until the nerve recovers. For simple contusions, treatment is RICE (see p.104), followed by natural remedies to speed up healing.

Fibular joint dysfunction

The two bones of the lower leg are jointed to each other just below the knee, on the outer side of the leg and at the ankle. These joints only allow small amounts of movement, but loss of that movement due to joint dysfunction can cause considerable problems.

Dysfunction may occur acutely due to a blow to the outside of the leg or an ankle sprain, or may come on more chronically due to long-term stresses such as regularly running around a banked track.

Pain at the upper joint is often confused with knee pain, as the two are so close, and because of this the real culprit is often missed. Pain at the lower joint may be diagnosed as an ankle sprain, particularly as the two could have occurred together.

A manual therapist skilled in manipulative diagnosis and treatment will be able to identify and treat the dysfunction.

"Tennis leg"

Tears of the **gastrocnemius** muscle at the back of the calf usually occur with sudden exertion of the calf, such as jumping or a sudden change of direction. They are more common in mature recreational athletes, and are often called "tennis leg."

Pain is immediate, and it is often described as feeling like being kicked in the calf. Some athletes also feel a "popping" sensation at the time of injury. Bruising may follow, and can be impressive. Attempting to raise up on the toes causes apprehension or actual pain. Treat with RICE, maintaining mobility by bending the unloaded ankle up and down within its pain-free range. After 48 hours, you should begin progressive stretching and strengthening exercises, always without pain. Adequate conditioning and a thorough warm-up is the key to prevention.

Compartment syndromes

The connective tissue, or fascia, divides the lower leg into four or five compartments, like the segments of an orange. Compartment syndrome is caused by an increase in pressure in one or more of these compartments, which prevents blood from draining out of the compartment(s), therefore leading to a further increase in pressure.

Chronic exertional compartment syndrome is a much more common chronic condition, where the increase in pressure is brought on by exercise and eases with rest. Increases in muscle size due to exercise may also contribute to the condition.

Pain will be felt within the whole of one or more of the compartments, and will run down much of the length of the lower leg, either toward the front or the back.

Treatment is initially rest and application of ice to reduce the pressure. Deep stretching of the fascia by a manual therapist may allow the compartments to increase in size, so reducing pressure.

If such a conservative approach does not improve the condition within six months, a surgeon could operate to split the compartments, in order to prevent pressure from building up.

ACUTE COMPARTMENT SYNDROMES

Acute compartment syndrome follows an injury that causes bleeding into a compartment. The symptoms are pain that continues to increase out of proportion to the initial injury and a tense, tender lower leg.

This is a surgical emergency, as failure to treat it within a few hours can result in permanent damage to the leg. Elevating the leg and applying ice to control the bleeding will, however, buy more time for the surgical team.

foot and
ankle
injuries

One quarter of all sports injuries presented for treatment involve the foot and ankle, with sprained ankles being the most common single sports injury of all.

FRACTURES AND DISLOCATIONS

Ankle fractures are quite common. The signs of pain, swelling, and difficulty bearing weight make for easy confusion with a severe sprain. Differentiating between the two requires medical attention.

Traumatic fractures of the foot may be the result of a collision, such as stubbing the toe, or dropping a heavy object on the foot. They can also be caused by forced movements beyond the normal range, as in an ankle sprain injury. These fractures are the result of the extreme movement, plus the contraction of muscles attempting to limit that movement. An avulsion fracture occurs when the muscle contraction pulls off a piece of the bone.

Signs of fracture are pain, tenderness, and swelling, and often an inability to bear weight. Treatment involves immobilization, which can range from taping for a simple toe fracture to casting or surgery for more serious injuries.

The foot is also a common site for stress fractures, as a result of repetitive impacts from running, particularly on hard surfaces.

Stress fractures present themselves as localized pain and tenderness on a bone, and may not be spotted on an X-ray until they begin to repair. Initial treatment is with RICE, followed by an avoidance of irritating actions and protection with hard-soled shoes. Immobilization is rarely needed.

"Soccer ankle"

Diffused pain and tenderness occurs on the front of the ankle from repeated stresses bending the foot downward. Kicking a ball hard with the top of the foot is a common cause. Repeated minor tears of the ligaments at the front of the ankle result in new bone growth, known as **osteophytes**, which interfere with the normal movement of the joint.

The application of ice and modifying activities to avoid extreme bends of the ankle can settle the symptoms. Soccer players have to kick the ball with the inside of the foot rather than the top. If this level of improvement and restriction of activity is acceptable, further treatment may not be necessary. Fully resolving the condition requires surgery to remove the new bone growth.

Ankle sprains

In 95 percent of cases, ankle sprains affect ligaments on the outer side of the ankle. Injuries occur when you "go over on your ankle" or land badly from a jump. Pain is immediate, and is followed quickly by swelling and, later, by bruising. Walking

The feet cope with enormous stresses as we accelerate or slow down while bearing our entire body weight.

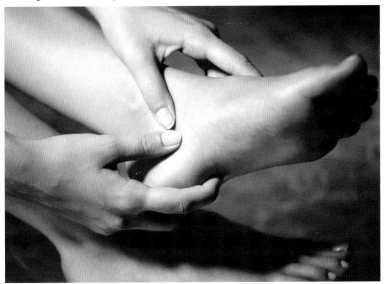

will be difficult, but if you cannot bear weight at all, suspect a fracture. You should apply RICE (see p.104) as soon after the injury as possible and avoid taking NSAIDs. A brace will help to support the ankle, while allowing you to flex and extend as much as you can without pain. The more severe the sprain, the more effective the brace needs to be to allow pain-free joint mobility.

Rehabilitation begins with isometric muscle contractions. When these are pain-free, progress to isotonic contractions, stretching, and functional exercises, such as using a wobble board (see rehabilitation beginning on p.138.) Functional rehabilitation is essential to return full function to the ankle complex and to prevent recurrent injuries.

Research has shown that even with complete rupture of the ligaments on the outer side of the ankle, recovery is faster, and as good, with non-surgical care as it is with surgical repair.

Severe injuries can also damage the ligaments that connect the lower ends of the tibia and fibula. If this junction becomes unstable, then surgery will probably be required. Symptoms that do not resolve as expected may indicate mechanical dysfunction caused by the original injury, which in turn could affect the joints of the foot and ankle or anywhere up to the lower back (or even higher). Other factors causing chronic symptoms are weakness of the peronial muscles on the outer side of the shin or instability of the ankle joint, which will require surgical reconstruction.

Achilles tendon injuries

Injuries affecting the Achilles tendon at the back of the ankle are often divided into tendonitis, tendon rupture, and Achilles bursitis.

Achilles "tendonitis" A presentation of pain, tenderness, and swelling of the Achilles tendon is often diagnosed as tendonitis, suggesting an inflammatory condition. The problem is far more likely to be **tendinosis**, indicating a degeneration or breakdown of normal tendon tissue. This differentiation is important because it influences the choice of treatment and rehabilitation.

A genuine tendonitis produces local warmth and often a "creaking" sensation in the tendon when the ankle is flexed and extended. This is due to inflammation of the outer part of the tendon or the surrounding sheath. In this case, anti-inflammatory remedies may be useful, and the condition could resolve itself relatively quickly.

In tendinosis, anti-inflammatory medication will not be beneficial and recovery will take several months, as the body has to rebuild the degenerated part of the tendon. Tendonitis and tendinosis may occur at the same time. Tendinosis is caused by overload or overuse, often exacerbated by problems in leg function, particularly tight calf and hamstring muscles.

Treatment requires reducing the load on the tendon, which often means stopping activities involving running or jumping. Heel lifts in shoes help reduce strain on the tendon further, and ice can be useful, even though there is no inflammation.

Dysfunction anywhere in the foot, leg, pelvis, or lower back can cause compensation that may focus stress on the Achilles. Calf stretching and strengthening within comfort stimulates the growth and alignment of fibers within the tendon. Expect the rehabilitation program to take three to six months.

Tendon rupture Rupture of the Achilles tendon is often the end result of an untreated tendinosis. Steroid injections have been used in the treatment of Achilles pain, based on the idea that the condition was inflammatory. Evidence is mounting, however, that these injections increase the risk of a tendon rupture. Ruptures manifest themselves as sudden pain at the back of the ankle, often with a "popping" sensation as the tendon snaps. Swelling follows, and there is an inability to raise up on the toes of the affected leg. Ruptures are more likely in the mature "weekend" athlete.

Choices of treatment are controversial, so ask your orthopaedic surgeon what the options are and what results they have achieved. Casting is often used, with or without surgical repair of the tendon.

Achilles bursitis The bursa between the Achilles tendon and the skin can be irritated by the heel of a shoe, and is sometimes referred to as a "pump bump." It announces its presence with localized pain and swelling where the shoe rubs on the tendon, which can develop into a callous.

Treatment is rest and the application of ice to control inflammation and pain. Heel lifts can reduce strain on the tendon to help speed recovery. You should also either change your shoes or modify your existing shoes by cutting a "V" out of the top of the heel, to remove the part that is pressing on the tendon. Ensure good function of the leg and foot as a whole, to reduce other possible causes of stress on the Achilles. Be particularly careful about shoes that have an "Achilles protector," as these high backs can make irritation much more likely. High-topped sports shoes need a low-cut back or plenty of room between the back of the shoe and your Achilles tendon.

Plantar fascitis

"The first few steps when I get up in the morning are agony. It's like having a marble under my heel." This is a classic description of plantar fascitis, or "triple jumper's heel." The pain is under the front of the heel, and deep probing will reveal an extremely tender point.

The plantar fascia is a strong cord running along the sole of your foot that helps to hold up the arch of the foot. If you think of the bony arch of the foot as being a bow, then the plantar fascia is the bowstring.

Repeated straining of the plantar fascia causes tiny tears where it attaches to the front of your heel bone, and it is this that causes the pain. It is more likely in mature athletes and in those who are overweight. Chronic cases can result in bone growth at the attachment to the heel bone showing up as a **heel spur** on X rays. However, heel spurs are also seen in people who have no problems with their plantar fascia.

Treatment is rest from irritating activities, such as running, and the use of ice to reduce inflammation. Heel lifts can reduce strain, and some have a special cut-out to reduce pressure on the sensitive area. Prescribed "orthotics" from a **podiatrist** can help ease strain while also helping to correct any underlying mechanical problems in the foot.

Deep friction massage will assist in resolving the problem, and any joint or muscle dysfunction should be corrected. Particular attention should be given to stretching the calf muscles (see p.101). Expect full recovery to take months rather than days or weeks. Steroid injections into the injury site have been used, but there is some evidence that these prolong the condition, so it is worth avoiding them.

Turf toe

This is a condition associated with playing sports on synthetic grass surfaces. Extreme bending of the big toe, as in setting off at a sprint, causes pain and swelling of the joint as ligaments are overstressed. The problem is more likely to occur if very flexible shoes are worn. Treatment is RICE, and taping the big toe so that it is bent down slightly, reducing strain on the joint while it recovers. A suitably qualified manual therapist can show you how to apply the tape. Use shoes with stiffer soles to take the strain off your toe.

Morton's neuroma

Pain in the webbed area between the bases of the toes is frequently caused by pressure on the nerve between the toes. The pain is sharp, occasionally running up the foot. Pressing the sides of the foot together will often reproduce the pain.

High heels and tight shoes are often the culprits, and low-heeled shoes, with space for the toes to wiggle, should be worn to reduce pressure on the nerve. Special supports or orthotics in the shoes can further reduce pressure, allowing the condition to settle. Severe unresponsive cases may benefit from surgery.

Skin problems

Athlete's foot Like all fungi, this infection likes warm, damp places and is most often seen between toes, where it causes peeling and fissuring of the skin. The skin is our first line of defense against infection, and broken skin can be an opening for a secondary infection. Treat by keeping the feet clean and dry, and by applying pure Tea Tree oil three or four times a day or by applying anti-fungal preparations.

Plantar warts Also known as "verrucas," these are the result of a viral infection, often contracted around swimming pools. Medical treatment includes chemical paints, freezing with liquid nitrogen, or cutting them out, but recurrence is common.

As with other kinds of warts, they often disappear spontaneously as the body develops immunity to the virus, so anything that improves your immune function is likely to speed up this process.

Black nail Bruising under the toenails is caused by trauma. Ensure your nails are not too long, and be meticulous in your choice of sports shoes. They must have enough room around the toes to prevent pressure on the nails, while being snug enough around the foot so that your feet do not slide forward in the shoe and bash your toes with each step.

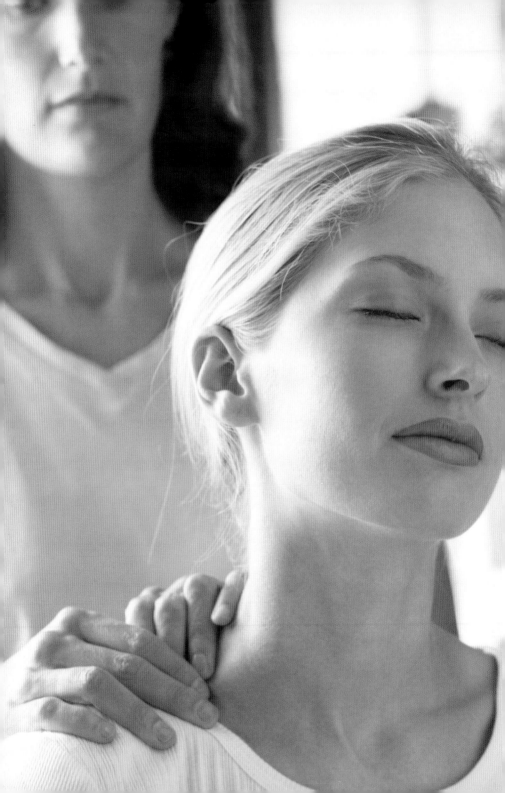

This section begins with advice on how to prevent injuries, as this is the best treatment strategy of all. This is followed by descriptions of the most useful therapies involved in the treatment of sports injuries. The color-coded tabs that appeared in Part One indicate which of these treatments are most useful for specific injuries.

The final part covers rehabilitation, explaining how to restore strength and function, both in the injured tissues and in the person as a whole.

ALL THE
options

PREVENTING

Professional decorators often claim that the results are "all in the preparation," and this is particularly true in injury prevention. The preparations you have made before you begin the performance of your sport have a major impact on your chances of remaining free from injury. There are several aspects of this preparation, ranging from training methods and warming-up to equipment selection, but they begin with the decision to play. Choosing your sport is the first step in the prevention process. Some people seem to have little choice at this point, their passion for a particular sport blinding them to any thought of the consequences. For the rest of us, however, there are some important points worth considering.

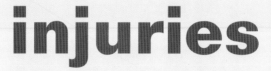

Consider your body

Different body types are more ideally suited to different types of activity. If you are short and broad, for example, you are likely to have short thick muscles and ligaments. You may suffer less injuries than someone with less robust tissues, but you are unlikely to achieve the extreme flexibility required to become a top-class gymnast. Look at the demands of the sport you are considering and then look at your physical characteristics, including your height, weight, strength, and flexibility. If you see any major mismatches, consider your choice with caution.

Some games, such as football, place extreme physical demands on the body, and require you to be very highly conditioned just to take part. These sports also produce high levels of injury, some of them serious, even in well prepared and skilled players. If you want to play sports in order to stay fit and have some fun, these sports may not be best suited to your purposes.

Start from where you are

The importance of starting small increases as we age, and is more significant for people who have been sedentary for long periods (for example, after an illness) or who have not exercised for several years. Even one hour a week of mild exercise increases your chances of a longer, disease-free life, and can be gradually increased to gain more of the benefits of exercise, including lower blood pressure and cholesterol levels.

Research shows that exercise benefits people with nearly every kind of disease known—even congestive heart failure. For those with a recent or current illness, however, it is necessary to exercise under the supervision of a healthcare practitioner. For more advice, see p.90.

Match your training to your sport

Does your sport require great muscular endurance or bursts of speed? Do you need great cardiovascular fitness or considerable flexibility? Different types of training produce different types of results, so make sure your training provides what you need to play your sport safely. (See p.94 for more guidance on which exercises do what.) For example, playing squash, which requires intense bursts of activity, will not prepare you for a half marathon, which requires sustained moderate effort. Therefore, you will not be preparing your body for, or learning the skills of, distance running.

general health
concerns

The state of your health before you start playing a sport should influence what sport you play and how you play it.

Do you need a checkup?

If it has been a long time since you did any exercise, and you have passed the first flush of youth, then a medical checkup is advisable. The more exercises you have

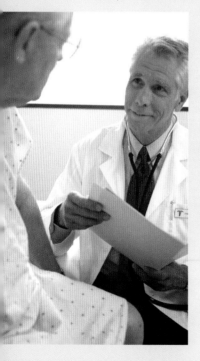

been involved in, the better you are likely to cope with a new sport. Yet even active people can develop high blood pressure, for example, which could go unnoticed without a physical. If in doubt, see your doctor.

People with a history of illness or injury would also be wise to seek advice before commencing a new sport. If you have had high blood pressure, heart problems, breathing difficulties, or conditions affecting your musculo-skeletal or nervous systems, you need to know that any new activity will not aggravate your condition.

Specific health concerns

There are also other health factors that require consideration. If you have undergone recent surgery,

Look at your sporting involvement in the context of your overall health, and select new activities that are appropriate for your current condition.

MEDICATIONS

- *Medications can interfere with sporting activity. Some drugs slow blood clotting, leading to the risk of excessive bleeding if you suffer an injury. Always check with your doctor or pharmacist.*
- *Increased activity can influence the effectiveness of your medication. Diabetics who use insulin may need to alter their dosage to cope with increased levels of activity.*
- *Some prescribed and over-the-counter medications can cause you to fail a drug test. Alternative medications that do not cause positive tests are usually available, so check with the governing body of your sport and your doctor.*

you should consult your surgeon before embarking on any new exercise. How long "recent" is depends on the surgery involved—it can vary from weeks to months.

Increasingly, surgeons are realizing that early activity tends to speed recovery for many patients. It is essential, however, that the activity is appropriate for the patient.

Warning signs

Physical exertion will cause breathlessness, but if this continues when you take a break, take it as a warning sign. A sore chest that is the result of a collision is a specific injury, but any unexplained chest pain is another matter entirely. Similarly, for any persistent abdominal pain, light-headedness, or dizziness you should go straight to a hospital or doctor's office. If you have an illness like a cold or cough, give your body the chance to recover from the illness before challenging it further.

A chronic illness may severely limit your activity but exercise will aid the treatment of many conditions. Those recovering from a heart attack or suffering with high blood pressure or depression can benefit from appropriate activity.

If you are severely overweight, exercise is a major way of improving your health, although some sports are more suitable than others. Running or other impact activities may place excessive strain on your joints, but aerobic fitness and fat burning can be more safely and comfortably achieved using non-impact exercises, like swimming, rowing, or cycling.

the mind-body
connection

While many of us have grown up in societies where the mind and body have been seen as separate entities, it is now well understood that this distinction is illusory. Every thought that you have produces changes in your body. Similarly, the state of your body influences your moods, and therefore the way in which you perceive the world.

Your attitude while playing sports not only influences your level of achievement and enjoyment, it can also affect your injury risk.

You are probably already aware that a lack of focus on what you are doing increases your chances of making silly mistakes. In the physically demanding environment of sports, such mistakes can lead to injury.

"Trying too hard" is another risk factor. While we all like to win, keep this in perspective with your overall purpose of playing sports for enjoyment. Focusing excessively on winning means that you are very likely to damage yourself in your struggle to win, and that you will be miserable every time you lose.

If you want sports to help you stay happy and healthy, make your sense of fun as strong as your muscles, and develop your sense of humor with your flexibility. Enjoy the actual playing at least as much as the score.

How much is connected?

The simple answer is: all of it. What happens if you start to think about a favorite food? See what it looks like, remember the smell, the way the texture feels in your mouth. Is your mouth watering yet? Think about that food long enough and it probably will be, and perhaps your stomach might begin to rumble, too. Simply thinking about food can produce physical responses in your body. Some yogis have developed this kind of mental control to a fine art, and are able to change heart rate, body temperature, and many other "unconscious" mechanisms at will.

Brain and body power

We usually associate thinking with the brain, as brain cells pass information among themselves by releasing chemicals known as neurotransmitters. However, it is now known that white blood cells also release and receive neurotransmitters, suggesting that they too are involved in "thinking." White blood cells rush to the site of an injury as part of the inflammatory response, so in a sense we could say that our "thinking" goes to the injury.

The enteric nervous system, or "abdominal brain," runs our digestive system. This has nearly as many nerve cells as the spinal cord, and carries out many of its functions without depending on the brain, so your digestive system does a lot of its "thinking" for itself. This gives a whole new meaning to following your "gut instinct."

Physical activities, such as exercise, also affect mental function. Exercise is a powerful tool to combat depression and the idea of a "runner's high" is now well known. The brain releases endorphins, or "happy chemicals," in response to exercise.

Rather than trying to list all of our body parts that are connected, it is easier to try and find a part of us that is unconnected.

What can the connection do?

When medical drugs are being tested, they are compared with a placebo, an inert pill that looks like the drug being tested. This is done to differentiate the effect of the drug from the placebo response, which causes people to get better because they believe that they are being treated.

Belief alone is enough to cause recovery in a significant number of cases. Even the most potent treatments produce their benefits by a combination of their actual effect and the placebo response.

In experiments, the powerful placebo of belief has even been able to overcome potent drugs, producing the opposite effect to that of the drug being taken. Disempowering beliefs can also inhibit or stop recovery, and in extreme cases cause perfectly healthy people to become sick and die (the so-called "voodoo death").

The placebo is a powerful component of any treatment plan, and this is why it is best to work with practitioners who are confident and optimistic about your ability to recover. Their confidence will rub off on you, improving your ability to achieve real health benefits.

Making use of the connection

How we think about things has as much impact as what we think about. Many people advocate "positive thinking," using tools such as repeated phrases or "affirmations." These can be useful, but what if your thoughts of "I will recover quickly... I will recover quickly..." meet thoughts of "Who are you trying to kid?"

The importance of believing For thoughts to have a positive impact, we must think of them in ways that are believable, so we need to understand how we believe things. You may think by creating visual images, and this is how most people answer questions like "what color is your front door?" You may create internal sounds, like thinking how your national anthem starts, or you may generate internal feelings, like remembering the sensation when you first dip your toe into a hot bath.

You don't have to actually see, hear, or feel these things to access the needed information, you just have to think them.

How you believe Let's look at this in a little more detail, so you can discover how you believe something. Think of something you absolutely believe to be true: your own address, that you love your children, or something else about which you have no doubt. As visual thinking is very popular, use a visual example. If you didn't think of an image, just imagine what it would have been like if you had.

Was the picture black and white or color? Was it still or moving? Was it bright or dull? How big is the picture when you think about it? How far away do you see the picture? In what direction? Is it clear or fuzzy?

Take time to think about this, and you will find that you code believable things by thinking about them in a very particular way. There is no right or wrong way to think, as we have all developed our own unique coding system. Now think about something you really don't believe at all, and notice the contrast in how you think about these two things.

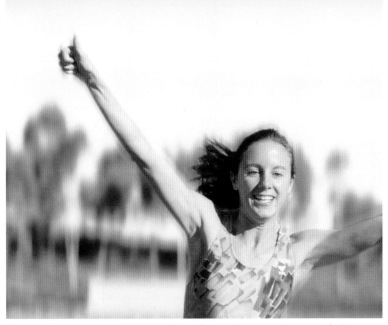

The way you choose to picture or hear things determines how you feel about them.

To develop a positive approach to your recovery, rather than trying to talk yourself into it, think about a positive recovery in a way that is believable to you.

Positive thinking Another example of this approach is the badminton player who had a knee injury. Once her knee recovered, her practitioner advised her to build its strength before going back onto the court. He suggested she start with some gentle jogging but she hated jogging.

The way she thought about badminton and how she thought about jogging was very different, so she was told to shift how she thought about jogging, to make it more like how she thought about badminton. She had to move the picture she thought of, increase the brightness, and make it sharper. When she had done this, she didn't feel so bad at the thought of jogging, and she can now jog happily whenever she needs to.

This way of working is just one of many developed by practitioners of Neuro Linguistic Programming, or NLP for short. If you would like help with issues involving motivation, strategies for acquiring new skills, or strategies for changing attitudes, it is recommended that you look into this system further.

training
principles

Training is a stimulus designed to produce a specific response from your body. The kind of training you should be doing depends on which aspect of performance you wish to affect. Different training methods are used to develop strength, power, muscular endurance, cardiovascular efficiency, flexibility, coordination, or specific skills. In the following chapters, we look at the variety of training methods used. Initially, however, it is important to consider the factors that apply to every training session.

Warm-up

Lack of warm-up is one of the most common causes of injury among recreational athletes. High-level athletes warm up not only to reduce the risk of injuries, but also to ensure they are performing at their peak level during the game.

The phrase "getting your second wind" describes the increased energy some athletes experience part way into the game, and this is actually the point at which they have warmed up. In other words, warming up properly means you have this level of energy right from the beginning of the game.

A good warm-up increases body temperature, making tissues more pliable and therefore less prone to injury by tearing. It also raises your heart rate and opens the small blood vessels that supply the muscles, so fuel and oxygen can be delivered more effectively. Athletes also have faster reaction times after warming up, leading to a more skilful performance.

To warm up effectively, progressively increase the level of activity of your large muscles, particularly those in your legs, hips, and buttocks. This can be done by starting with gentle jogging, gradually building up the pace and complexity of your activity as you warm-up.

Repeatedly go through the motions of your sport, initially without any speed or power. Apart from warming your body up, you can also use this time to consciously practice and refine your skills, without any pressure to perform in a real game.

Just five or ten minutes warm up will mean you start your activity in a much more prepared state, both mentally and physically.

Cool down

Gradually reducing activity after vigorous exercise prevents blood from pooling in muscles, so waste products are removed more effectively, reducing the chance of muscle soreness.

Stretching is the ideal way to do this, and you can make more progress in your flexibility training by stretching when your muscles are warm.

Coaching and form

Exercise stresses the body; however, the stress has to be at a level appropriate to your sport, and to your level of fitness and physical condition, otherwise it is just another way of creating injuries. Performing exercises using good posture and alignment, and making the correct movements at the right pace, is described as exercising with good form. To attain and maintain good form requires guidance from someone who knows what constitutes good form, and a degree of concentration on your part.

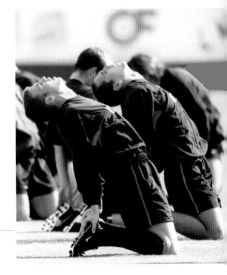

Find a qualified coach or fitness trainer who can teach you the skills needed for the safe performance of your sport, along with training exercises. This will enable you to get more fun out of your sport.

An effective warm-up can ensure peak performance as well as protection from injury.

get **fit** for
sports

You don't play sports to get fit, you get fit to play sports. While playing sports may increase your fitness, you need at least a basic level of fitness to play safely. Once your are fit, sports will contribute toward maintaining that fitness.

A key area of fitness you need in most sports is cardio-vascular endurance—the ability of your heart and lungs to deliver oxygenated blood to your muscles. Increased cardio-vascular endurance comes as a result of making your heart muscle stronger, and increasing the number of small blood vessels or capillaries supplying blood to your muscles.

Aerobic and anaerobic exercise

Muscles work by burning fuel either aerobically or anaerobically. Aerobic means "with air," with the oxygen needed to burn fuel being supplied in adequate amounts by your heart and lungs. Burning fuel aerobically is the most efficient form of exercise, and it also has the advantage of encouraging the burning of fat. Anaerobic burning of fuel is less efficient and produces a buildup of wastes in the muscle. These wastes, such as lactic acid, cause the muscles to fatigue, and if levels become high enough the muscles stop working altogether. To exercise aerobically, limit the intensity of the exercise, so you do not exceed your capacity to deliver oxygen to your muscles. Moderate activity that you can sustain, such as jogging, is aerobic exercise, while intense activity, like sprinting or weight lifting, is anaerobic exercise.

Increasing cardiovascular fitness

The greater your cardiovascular fitness, the more intensely you can exercise before

Aerobe Zone

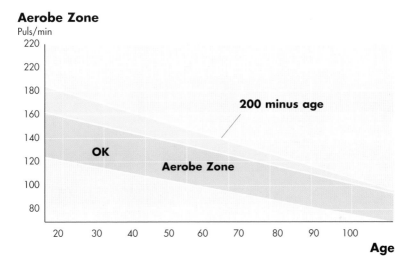

Puls/min

shifting into anaerobic fuel burning. This means your exercise capacity will increase, which is helpful in almost every sport. Greater cardiovascular fitness produces many of the health benefits associated with regular exercise, including lowering high blood pressure and reducing the risk of a heart attack.

To increase your cardiovascular endurance, you need to exercise so that you raise your heart rate sufficiently to stimulate your body to become fitter (but not so high that it becomes dangerous). Your training must get you into this **target heart rate zone**, and keep you there for a sustained period of time. This must be done frequently—a reasonable rule of thumb would be 20–60 minutes of exercise, three to five days per week.

Appropriate activities include brisk walking, jogging, swimming, and cycling. The above graph gives you an average indication of target zones relative to age. If you have not exercised for a while, aim at the lower end of your zone, gradually moving up as your fitness increases.

To monitor your heart rate while you are exercising, use two or three fingers (but not the thumb, which has a pulse of its own) to check your pulse—either on the thumb side of the front of your wrist or on the front of your neck just to the side of your windpipe. Practice this until you can find your pulse easily. Count the beats for 15 seconds. Multiply the number by four to get your heart rate in beats per minute. Alternatively, use a heart rate monitor, available from sports equipment retailers.

safety

measures

Preparing yourself for your sport is an essential part of injury prevention. It is also vital that the facilities around you are also prepared, in order for you to safely enjoy your activity.

Temperature

An advantage of being mammals is that we can regulate our body temperature, but this does have its limits. Outdoor activities in extremely cold conditions, such as skiing, can push us beyond our limits, leading to hypothermia and frostbite. Always ensure you have adequate protection against the cold, and heed warnings when conditions are so severe that activities need to be postponed.

Sometimes even indoor conditions are too cold for your planned activity. Whether this is due to poor planning or heating failure, wear more layers while you warm up, shedding them only when you are maintaining your temperature.

Exercise generates heat, which can be a problem in hot climates, as we can overheat. The evaporation of perspiration is a major cooling mechanism, but this becomes less efficient the higher the humidity, thus placing us at greater risk from heat illnesses. In hot conditions, drink more water than you think you need, and keep drinking frequently to replace water lost as perspiration.

Exercise-induced sweating routinely causes fluid loss of between three to four pints (one-and-a-half to two liters) of water per hour, rising to six pints (three liters) per hour under extreme conditions. If this water loss is not replaced, you become dehydrated, impairing both your physical and mental performance.

Continuing to exercise and generate heat beyond our ability to cool ourselves can lead to heat exhaustion and, eventually, the potentially fatal heatstroke. Should you begin to suffer from muscle cramps, nausea, headaches, dizziness, or weakness, you should stop the activity at once, drink plenty of water and lower your body temperature with cool compresses.

Physical environment

Look out for potential risks in the area in which you will be playing. This could include broken glass on fields, spillages causing slippery indoor surfaces, and obstructions around the playing area.

Lack of hygiene, particularly in changing areas, increases the spread of infections, such as athlete's foot and plantar warts. If the facilities are dirty, let the person responsible know that conditions are not acceptable.

Equipment

In many sports, people underestimate the injury risk caused by poor or inappropriate equipment. Safety doesn't often require the latest, most expensive equipment, but it does require equipment that is suited both to you and the sport you are involved in. It must be in good enough condition to fulfill its function and, if appropriate, be adjusted for your needs.

People often use equipment that is designed for one sport while participating in another. Modern sports shoes are often designed for specific sports, and are ill suited for others. For example, squash shoes are not designed for the shock-absorbing job of running. Correcting certain problems may be as simple as putting an extra layer of wrap on your racket handle, so it is the right size for you, or recognizing that running shoes have a finite lifespan and replacing them when necessary.

Supervision

Some sports require supervision, whether it be in the form of a lifeguard, a referee, or a coach or instructor. Those people who lead groups in outdoor adventure sports, such as white-water rafting, mountaineering, or alpine skiing, often have to fill several of these roles.

In all cases, it is important to make sure that the supervisors are suitably qualified, with a good understanding not just of the techniques of the sport, but also of the risk factors and appropriate actions to take in an emergency.

Check that there is an adequate level of supervision for the number of people involved. If safety or first aid equipment is needed, find out who provides it and who knows how to use it.

exercises

In addition to cardiovascular endurance, exercises can be used to increase strength, power, muscular endurance, and flexibility. When designing a training program, it is important to choose exercises that match your needs.

How much strength do you need?

Resistance exercises, such as weight training and push-ups, are used to strengthen muscles. Even in obvious strength sports, such as weight lifting or shot put, it is not so much strength that is needed, but power.

Strength is the ability to move a load, but power is the ability to accelerate that load. Resistance training against a relatively high load, through a full range of movement for the muscles involved, tends to increase the ability to generate power.

If you play badminton or practice aerobic dance, you may not think you have a high demand for power. However, every time you make a quick change in direction, your muscles have to rapidly apply the brakes to stop the momentum of your whole body, before quickly accelerating it in another direction.

In Part One: Understanding Your Sports Injury, "rapid changes in direction" were repeatedly described as a likely cause of many injuries. Often this is because muscles are not strong enough to cope with the loads placed on them.

Muscular endurance, the ability to keep on applying power, is also required in many sports. Resistance training (see below) with moderate loads, when performed for a high number of repetitions, stimulates the muscle to build further endurance.

Resistance training

Resistance training often takes the form of weight training, whether with free weights or the great variety of machines now available in gyms. Floor exercises that use your own body weight for resistance and systems using "rubber bands" to provide resistance are other options.

The most important aspect of safe and effective resistance training is good form. Many injuries are caused by doing exercises badly. Common errors include poor positioning, jerking with the load, and trying to use too heavy a load.

Many people do exercises dangerously, using completely inappropriate movements, because they are trying to impress themselves or others with the loads they are using. Get a qualified trainer to design a program for you and to teach you how to do each exercise safely. A good trainer will check on you periodically, ensuring that you are progressing safely and are not developing any bad habits.

There are several ways to make resistance exercises harder, without increasing the weight. You can increase the number of repetitions, move the load more quickly (but still smoothly), or move the load very slowly.

You do not get stronger during training sessions. Your muscles increase in strength while recovering from a training session. Adequate rest between training sessions is vital if you want to improve. Training too frequently impedes progress and increases your risk of injury.

The importance of mobility

Healthy muscles are both strong and flexible. Stiff muscles are more liable to injury, and they can also limit movement so you cannot perform the movements of your sport properly. Tight tissues within the body can also have a detrimental effect on many areas of general health, inhibiting movements such as breathing, impeding blood flow, and wasting energy as you work to overcome their resistance.

Practicing exercises with good form increases their effectiveness and reduces the risk of injuries.

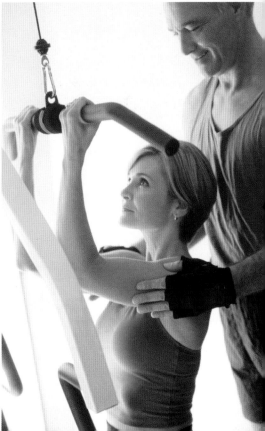

THE PRINCIPLES OF STRETCHING EXERCISES

As with resistance training, correct form is vital for safe and efficient stretching. Incorrect form can at best render stretches ineffective and at worst can stress joints, causing injury.

Heeding the following points will help you get the most out of your stretching routine.

■ Pay careful attention to all the details of form when learning and practicing stretching exercises.

■ To increase your range of movement, many stretches may need to be sustained for 30 seconds or more.

■ Breathe slowly and deeply, and focus on relaxing the muscles being stretched. You should feel a sense of stretch in the muscles you are working on. However, you should not feel any pain, and you should not feel strain in any joint. Think in terms of your body lengthening to produce a stretch.

You can increase the effect of stretching exercises using a method known as post-isometric relaxation. This approach is derived from the muscle energy techniques used by many manual therapists (see p.111 for further information).

■ Take the muscle involved to its comfortable limit of stretch.

■ While holding this position, contract the stretched muscle as if you are trying to shorten it again. It is very important that no movement occurs. Maintain this moderate contraction for 10 seconds. Ten to twenty percent of a full strength contraction is all that is required.

■ Relax the muscle, then gently stretch to its new limit. You will normally be able to increase the stretch by several small steps using this simple method.

Contracting a muscle, without any movement occurring, is classed as an **isometric contraction**, and is an essential component of this technique.

Specific stretching exercises

The following stretching exercises are for different regions of the body. Together they make up a general stretching program. You may need to add other exercises to deal with particular problems, or for the needs of specific sports, so consult your practitioner or trainer for guidance.

Practice each of these stretches for at least 30 seconds.

Neck

Forward bend Stand or sit upright, and consciously relax your shoulders so that they drop outward away from your ears. As you breathe in, feel your spine lengthen upward. As you breathe out, let your head drop forward, so your chin goes down toward your chest. With each breath out, allow the weight of your head to drop further forward.

Side bend Start as you did for the previous exercise. Relax. As you keep your face facing forward—a mirror may help here—drop your right ear toward your right shoulder. Leave your right shoulder relaxed. (It can be useful to place an imaginary bag of sand on the left shoulder at this point, as gravity lowers both the head and left shoulder, so the neck muscles between are stretched.) Repeat the process on the other side.

head turn

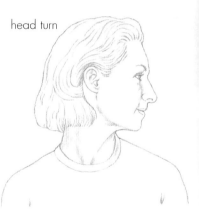

Head turn Allow the top of your head to float up effortlessly and your shoulders to relax. Turn your head as far to the right as you can without straining. Keeping your head in this position, relax your shoulders even further. Imagine them going wider and lower. Repeat this on the other side.

Back

Standing side bend Stand upright with your feet pointing forward, shoulder-width apart or a little wider.

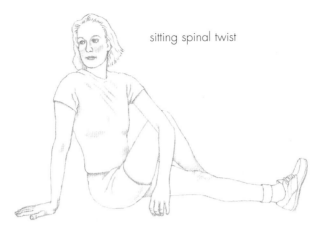

sitting spinal twist

Bend to your right side, sliding your right middle finger down the side of your leg, where the seam of your trousers would be. To make sure you are staying straight, stand with your heels an inch (2.5 cm) from a wall and let the tips of both shoulder blades glide along the wall as you bend.

Hang in this position, letting the weight of your body gently stretch the muscles at the side of your back and hip. This is a good stretch for the quadratus lumborum muscle. Repeat on the other side.

Sitting forward bend Sit toward the front of an upright chair with your feet flat on the floor, a little more than shoulder-width apart. Make sure your knees are directly above your feet. Allow your spine to lengthen as your head floats upward.

Let your head bend forward taking your chin toward your chest. Continue bending forward by rolling down the whole of your spine. As your flexibility develops, your upper body will end up going between your knees. Relax, allowing your body to "hang." Come up again by gradually "unrolling" your spine, until you are upright once more.

Sitting spinal twist This simplified yoga exercise stretches your spine into rotation and also stretches your piriformis muscle on the bent leg side. The instructions may appear complicated, but the picture (above) will help you to see that this is a simple exercise.

Sit as tall as you can on the floor, with both legs out straight in front of you. If this is difficult, put your hands on the floor behind you to keep your upper body lengthened rather than slumped. Bend your right knee so that the sole of your right foot is flat on the floor beside your left knee. Now lift your right foot over your left knee, so that it is flat on the floor next to the outside of your left knee.

Put the side of your left elbow on the outside of your bent right knee and your right hand on the floor behind you. Gently pushing your left elbow against your knee helps you to turn your upper body to the right, while keeping your bent right knee over your left leg.

With each breath in, feel your spine lengthen; with each breath out, feel yourself turn a little further. Repeat the process on the other side.

Hips

Hip flexor stretch Kneel in an erect position, then put your right foot flat on the floor in front of you.

While keeping your spine lengthened, bend your right knee, allowing your hips to go down toward the floor. There is a tendency here to hollow your lower back— resist this by concentrating on dropping your tailbone down toward the floor.

In the stretching position, your right knee should be vertically above your right foot. If it isn't, adjust the position of your right foot. You may need a pad under your left knee for comfort.

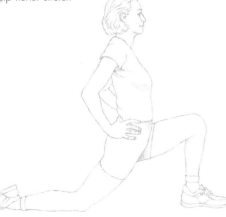

ip flexor stretch

Concentrate on lengthening your spine so that the top of your head goes up and your tailbone goes down. You should feel the stretch in your left groin, or on the front of your left thigh, not in your back. Repeat on the opposite side.

Hip adductor stretch Stand with your feet wide apart and toes pointing forward. Turn your right foot out 45 degrees. Keeping your upper body upright, bend your right knee so that it goes over your right foot. Your knee should not go past your foot and your shin should be vertical.

Keep your left knee straight by contracting your quadriceps on the front of your thigh. This protects your knee from lateral strain. Keep both feet flat on the floor. The stretch should be felt on the inside of your left thigh. Repeat on the other side.

Knees

Quadriceps stretch Stand with your feet together and your left hand on a wall or piece of furniture in front of you for balance.

Bend your right knee, and take hold of your right foot with your right hand behind you. If this is difficult, hold onto a belt or scarf looped around your ankle.

Keep your spine long, avoid arching your lower back by dropping your tailbone toward the floor. Use a mirror to check that your hips are level. Draw your right foot toward your right buttock, while keeping your right knee close to your left.

Feel the stretch on the front of your right thigh or hip. Repeat on the other side.

Hamstring stretch It is important with hamstring stretches to make sure you are focusing on the hamstrings and not the lower back. You will need a belt or scarf.

Lie on your back and bend your right knee up toward your chest. Hold an end of the scarf in each hand and loop it around the sole of your foot. Your right hip may tend to hitch up toward your shoulder, so make sure that both sides of your waist stay lengthened.

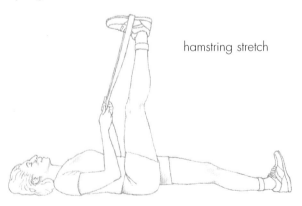

hamstring stretch

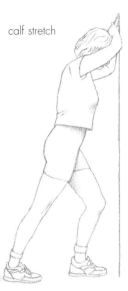

calf stretch

Slowly straighten your right knee, so that your right foot goes upward. Once you reach your comfortable limit, concentrate on relaxing your right hamstring. Repeat on the other side.

Calf

Standing calf stretch Stand facing a wall or door, so you can just touch it with your fingertips. Step forward, placing your left foot close to the wall, and lean your hands and forearms on the wall. Make sure that the outside of your right foot is at right angles to the wall, so your foot will be turned slightly inward.

Bend your left knee, so that your hips drop forward. Your body should make a straight line from your right heel to your shoulders. Lengthen your right heel away from you, as if it were sinking into the floor. You should feel a comfortable stretch in your right calf or in the back of your knee. Repeat this on the other side.

Shoulders

"Face of the cow" exercise Stand upright with a scarf or belt hanging from your right hand. Stretch your right arm upward and outward, then bend the elbow so that your right hand goes down behind your head. The scarf should then hang down your back.

"face of the cow"

Stretch your left arm downward and outward, then bend the elbow so your left hand goes behind your waist. Catch hold of the scarf with your left hand.

Creep your hands along the scarf toward each other, until you reach your comfortable limit. Lengthen your spine, so that your lower back has a normal gentle curve (not excessively arched) and your neck is straight.

Feel your right elbow lengthening up and back, and your left elbow lengthening down and back. Repeat this on the other side.

TREATING

This section covers the steps to take at the time an injury occurs. This may be something to do for yourself, but if others are involved in your sport, agreeing how you might cooperate in advance will make dealing with injuries easier and more effective. This could be as simple as each of you knowing where the first aid equipment is kept and how to use it. Obviously, at the time of an injury you may not be very mobile, so having someone else who can get you a ice pack, or make a phone call, can make a huge difference. The first section of this book suggested the practitioners who are likely to be most helpful in dealing with particular injuries. Yet even within a single profession, you will come across a variety of styles and approaches used by individual practitioners, so you need to know who to go to.

injuries

Picking your team

If you were picking a sports team to play with, you would ideally choose players who were competent at the sport, confident of their abilities, good communicators, pleasant company, and who had a proven track record. Picking your treatment team based on the same criteria will stand you in good stead.

Competence Looking for practitioners who are well qualified is made easier with those professions that have formal registration. These professions usually have listings of qualified practitioners, so you can find someone in your area. Their members will be identifiable by a title or specific letters after their names.

Within professions, there may also be special interest groups, with a particular interest in treating sports injuries. This is often the case within the manual therapies, for example. Talking to other athletes who have had similar injuries can be useful, as they will often recommend therapists they found particularly helpful.

Confidence Don't be afraid to discuss your injury with practitioners before making an appointment. They won't be able to diagnose your problem over the telephone, but you will be able to get an impression of how they will deal with you.

A practitioner should inspire your confidence. While a realistic approach to your recovery and rehabilitation may involve commitment over a significant period of time, you should avoid anyone who takes an overly pessimistic view of your injury.

Unfortunately, some serious injuries may mean that you should avoid some sports. While this does not condemn you to a life of inactivity, it may mean you have to change to a new sport or modify your existing one. If injury limits your usual sport, your practitioner should have a positive attitude, encouraging you to try different activities that you can safely enjoy.

Personality It is important that you feel comfortable with your practitioners, talking, asking questions, and receiving answers you understand. In general, an encounter with your practitioner should leave you feeling positive. If you are going to be working with more than one practitioner, they need to be able to communicate effectively with one another. The ideal is to have a team that is working in an integrated manner to achieve a common goal—your optimal recovery and return to activity.

immediate
first aid

Taking the right action at the time of an injury can have
a significant impact on your subsequent recovery.
Appropriate action stops the injury from getting worse,
limits tissue damage, and speeds your recovery, thus
reducing the long-term consequences.

General first-aid procedures are outside the scope of this book, but you should
become familiar with them. By practicing first-aid techniques at a first-aid course,
you are far more likely to remember them in an emergency.

RICE

There is one key first-aid approach that is vital for a wide variety of sports injuries.
RICE stands for Rest, Ice, Compression, and Elevation. This should be your initial
response to all sprains, strains, and other soft tissue injuries.

Rest First stop your activity, as you need to give yourself time to check if everything
is alright. If you felt a mild, instantaneous pain, which disappeared immediately,
carefully and slowly repeat the motion you were making to see if the pain occurs
again. If not, repeat the motion again with slightly more vigor. If there is still no
discomfort, gradually build up the intensity of your activity until you are back to
playing level. Stop if you have any recurrent pain, joint dysfunction, swelling, or
bruising. Playing through the pain can turn a small tear into a big tear and a big
tear into a complete rupture.

Ice This refers to cooling the site of an injury. Cold causes blood vessels to contract,
so there is less blood flow into the area. Reducing the flow reduces the amount of

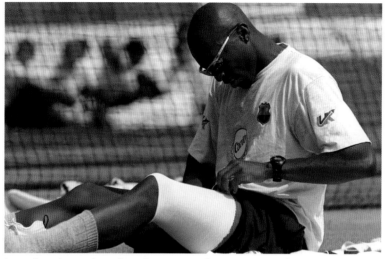

Immediate first aid can limit the severity of an injury.

bleeding from damaged tissues, and makes it easier for the body to produce a clot to prevent further blood loss. Cold also numbs the area, so it produces an immediate local pain reducing effect. Cold can be applied by using a proprietary ice pack or a plastic bag containing a mixture of water and ice.

Compression on an injury reduces bleeding and swelling. Elastic bandages are a simple and very adaptable way of providing compression. They can also hold a ice pack over the injury.

Make sure bandages are not too tight, as they can impair circulation. Fingers or toes going cold, or turning purple or white, indicate that bandages are too tight. Apply compression around, rather than just at, the site of the injury. For example, a bandage on a knee should extend part way down the calf and part way up the thigh.

Elevation Raising the injured area reduces fluid pressure, and is another way to help limit bleeding and swelling. If you have injured your knee, for example, sit or lie down with your knee propped up on a chair or bench. Making yourself comfortable aids relaxation, which helps in the repair process.

medications

Some medications are used frequently in the treatment of sports injuries, but many authorities have questioned their effectiveness and safety.

Non-steroidal anti-inflammatory drugs (NSAIDs)

These are often the first line drugs in the treatment of both acute and chronic injuries, and include drugs such as aspirin, ibuprofen, naproxen, and diclofenac. The idea behind the use of these drugs is that the inflammatory response causes much of the pain, so reducing the inflammation is seen as beneficial.

However, current evidence suggests that the anti-inflammatory effect of these drugs is minimal in injuries, and many healthcare practitioners advise against them in such cases. They all have pain killing properties, and it appears to be these that reduce symptoms. Studies demonstrate that they may be no more effective than ordinary pain killers (analgesics), and they do not alter the pattern of recovery. There also appears to be no evidence of their benefit in the treatment of chronic injuries. Studies show that they are no better than plain analgesics or placebos. There is mounting concern that NSAIDs may impair the healing of damaged cartilage, suggesting that they may make some joint injuries worse. This questionable effectiveness must also be seen in light of the risks associated with this class of drugs.

The main side effect of these drugs is irritation of the digestive tract. This may produce discomfort, and can cause ulceration and bleeding. The development of an ulcer may not produce symptoms until the ulcer perforates the digestive tract. Lack of a history of ulcers is no proof of safety. Overall, NSAIDs are responsible for many deaths every year. NSAIDs may aggravate asthma and can also impair blood clotting mechanisms, so should not be used if bleeding still occurs.

Corticosteroids

These are derived from the hormone cortisone and, unlike NSAIDs, they have definite, powerful anti-inflammatory effects. They are usually used in the form of injections, directly to the site of an injury. They can have dramatic symptom-relieving power, especially for chronic tendonitis and ligament strain, but again, their use is questionable. Corticosteroids should not be used in acute injuries, as stopping inflammation prevents healing from taking place.

In chronic injuries, there is no point using them unless inflammation is present, yet they are used in the treatment of tennis elbow, rotator cuff injuries, and Achilles tendon injuries—all conditions where investigations reveal no inflammation.

There are also risks associated with these "steroid injections." Corticosteroids are catabolic steroids, which means they encourage the breaking down of tissue. The use of corticosteroid injections into tendons or ligaments increases the risk of tendinosis. Safer injections target the tissue surrounding the site of the injury.

Counter irritants

These are creams or gels to rub on your skin over the site of an injury that stimulate the skin. Nerve impulses from the skin travel through fast nerve fibers and reach the "gate" in the spinal cord before the slower pain signals, where they then block the transmission of pain. Counter irritants can be extremely effective.

Medications may relieve symptoms, but are they supporting healing?

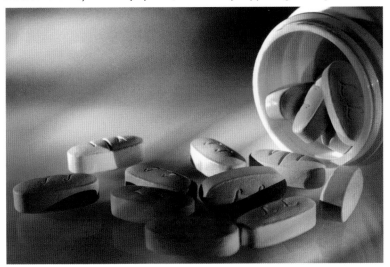

manual
therapies

These are the "hands-on" therapies, such as osteopathy, chiropractic, physiotherapy, and massage. They take a physical approach to treating physical dysfunction, such as weak or tight muscles and stiff joints.

Physical treatment can produce benefits through a variety of mechanisms. Seeing how these therapies work will help you to understand why your therapist does what he or she does, and what results you can expect from the treatment.

The aims of treatment

Restore movement Making tight muscles flexible and stiff joints mobile is perhaps the most obvious of outcomes for manual treatment. Successful treatment is often immediately apparent, as most therapists will measure mobility before and after treatment. This measurement need only be as simple as seeing how far you can turn your head or how far you can reach your hand up your back.

Improve fluid flow Every cell in your body relies for its health on the flow of fluids, delivering nutrition and removing waste. Proper movement of blood, lymph, and intercellular fluids is also essential for the transmission of your body's chemical messengers, such as hormones, as well as for the delivery of medications. Impaired flow can be improved by manual treatment.

Normalize nervous messages The organization of normal movement depends on the appropriate messages flashing around the nervous system at incredible speeds. Any abnormality in this communication leads to dysfunction. Strains and injuries can

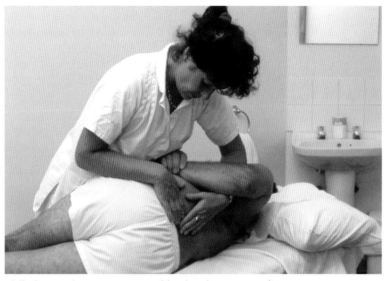

Skilled manual treatment can aid healing by restoring function.

lead to irritation in the nervous system, either leading to too many messages being sent or to messages not reaching their destination.

Some of the treatment methods used by manual therapists are specifically intended to restore normality to nervous communication, thus re-establishing normal movement function.

Improve coordination Injury may be caused by poorly coordinated movement or it may produce coordination problems. Some treatment methods are designed to help restore or improve coordination, and these are often part of the rehabilitation program.

These methods may include the use of simple equipment, such as wobble boards to improve ankle function and balance, or rely on progressively more challenging exercises to rebuild skills appropriate to your sport.

Restoring or improving coordination is vital to enable a full return to sports activity and to reduce the risk of reinjury. Coordination is dependent on the integrated function of mind and body. Use of the postural therapies introduced on p.132 aids the development of coordination.

DIAGNOSING THE PROBLEM

Before appropriate treatment can begin, your practitioner needs to gain an understanding of the nature of your injury and the factors that caused it. The extent of the diagnostic process will depend on your practitioner. You might expect a more extensive examination from a primary care provider, such as an osteopath or chiropractor, than from a massage therapist. The following factors are the typical elements of an extensive diagnostic investigation.

- *The first step is taking a thorough history, including details of the onset of the injury, and any other factors that may have contributed to the injury or may interfere with its healing. Ideally, this should include details of your medical history, use of medications, occupation, and leisure activities.*
- *You should also be asked about factors that aggravate or relieve your symptoms, such as particular positions, movements, or activities.*
- *The examination may cover standard medical tests, such as checking your blood pressure or listening to your heart, along with X rays or Magnetic Resonance Imaging (MRI) scans (see p.137).*
- *Observation of your posture and a simple range of movement tests should follow, before moving onto a more detailed examination of the injured or dysfunctional tissues.*
- *The practitioner will be testing muscles and joints by observation or palpation. Palpation is the art of gaining information through the sense of touch, and is a skill that is highly developed in the training of a skilled manual therapist. The palpating hand can detect subtle changes in tissue tension, temperature, degree of swelling, and smoothness of joint movements.*
- *Your muscles and joints will be assessed for their integrity and mobility. This is likely to include checking muscle strength as well as the range and quality of the movement of joints.*

Available methods

There is a wide range of different treatment methods available to the manual therapist. Which ones are used will depend on the training and preferences of the individual therapist. There are some general differences between the professions, and these are covered in the text on specific therapies.

Similar methods may be referred to by different names, depending on the profession of the practitioner. The following categories of treatment methods have therefore been listed using simple descriptive names. Some of the more well-known names your practitioner may use are also included.

"Massage" techniques These techniques often utilize pressing, stroking, or kneading. They are the basis of massage therapy, but in highly specific forms they are used extensively by many physiotherapists and osteopaths. They may be referred to as "soft tissue techniques" or "neuromuscular techniques." Practitioners of orthopedic medicine utilize deep transverse friction massage.

Contract and stretch techniques Muscle relaxation is increased after an isometric contraction—a contraction without movement. These techniques are used therapeutically to stretch contracted muscle and to restore normal joint mobility.

The practitioner places the muscle in a position of comfortable stretch. You then contract lightly against the stretch for a few seconds while the practitioner resists. Relaxation after the contraction usually allows you to reach a greater degree of stretch. Osteopaths refer to these as "muscle energy techniques," while physiotherapists often call them "proprioceptive neuromuscular facilitation," or PNF for short.

You can use these methods yourself to increase the effectiveness of your own stretching program—see the exercises on p.96.

Rhythmic techniques These involve applying a gentle rhythmic stretch to improve mobility. It is a traditional approach in osteopathy, where it is known as "articulation," while physiotherapists refer to it as "mobilization techniques."

A quick click This is the most memorable of techniques, as it seems to be the most dramatic. You are carefully positioned, then a rapid but very short, controlled movement is applied by the practitioner, which is often accompanied by a "pop" or "click" as the joint regains full mobility. The experience is not painful, and many patients find the experience pleasant because of the immediate sense of release felt.

Many chiropractors utilize these rapid techniques extensively, or even exclusively, terming them "adjustments." Osteopaths refer to "high velocity thrust," but generally use them as just one option in treating dysfunction. A minority of physiotherapists are trained to use "mobilization with impulse." There are, however, a few circumstances in which these techniques should not be used, such as joint instability, and your practitioner should screen you for these. In the hands of a well-trained practitioner, these techniques are both safe and effective.

Positional release techniques Originating from the discoveries of American osteopath Dr. Lawrence Jones, these techniques hold strained tissues in a position of maximum ease, to allow relaxation to occur. Jones termed these "strain-counter strain" techniques. Several variations on the theme have sprung up since, and practitioners from any of the professions may have trained in them.

Deactivating trigger points These points are a common and often missed cause of pain. They are tender little nodules, usually within a muscle, that cause referred symptoms. They can be produced by a traumatic injury, but are more often the result of long-term strain. Nutritional deficiencies can also be a contributory factor. Symptoms of pain, and sometimes pins and needles, will be worse when the affected muscle is stretched, loaded, or exposed to the cold.

Diagnosis requires a therapist who is aware of trigger points, and picks up clues from the patterns of pain and the movements that increase symptoms. A variety of methods can deactivate a trigger point, including pressure, cooling, muscle energy techniques, positional release, acupuncture, or infrared light therapy. Deactivation is followed by stretching to restore normal muscle length.

Photonic stimulation

This treatment uses a photonic stimulator, which produces infrared light that penetrates the skin to promote increased blood flow and circulation to damaged or compromised parts of the body. The stimulator is directed on traumatized nerves, acupuncture or trigger points, and restores normal function to the tissues. First, the function of the nerves is restored, then blood circulation returns to the affected area bringing oxygen and nutrients as well as removing waste.

Photonic therapy is a natural therapy promoting the body's own immune and healing responses without the need for needles or drugs. The treatment can help with sports injuries as well as a range of other health problems, from ulcers and rheumatism to chronic fatigue.

Managing your recovery

It is vital for you to know how to speed recovery and prevent recurrences. Advice that you are given is likely to include the prescription of exercises, modification of training programs, and advice on ergonomics in work or leisure activities.

Osteopathy

Osteopathy originated in 1874 and was created by Dr. Andrew Taylor Still of Kirksville, Missouri. Still became disillusioned with the medical practices of his day, particularly when he lost his wife and three of his children during an outbreak of meningitis. He set out to find a better way to treat illness and injury, by going back to the study of the human body. This was a radical step, considering that the accepted treatments of the time included bleeding, purging, and "heroic" dosing with highly toxic "medicines."

Qualifications Osteopaths require a five-year doctorate degree, equivalent to the training of a medical doctor. Osteopaths are D.O.s, or Doctors of Osteopathy. They have the same scope of practice as medical doctors (M.D.s), including being able to prescribe drugs and perform surgery. The key difference is the exposure to osteopathic philosophy and the training in osteopathic manipulative techniques.

Principles Unlike many healthcare systems, osteopathy has clear principles on which osteopaths base their work.

The body is a whole. Osteopaths understand the integrated nature of the body and its function, recognizing that dysfunction in one area will impact the function of other areas. Osteopaths always consider the whole person, including the psychological makeup, whatever apparently specific injury has occurred. For example, that nagging hip pain may be due to the stresses focused on the hip by the dropped arch on your foot, which in turn are compounded by your depressed state.

The body has self-regulating and self-repairing mechanisms. While this observation may seem obvious, many healthcare practices seem to ignore it. Osteopaths work with your natural healing mechanisms, by removing obstacles to the normal functioning of the body on which they depend.

Structure and function are interrelated. The structural organization of the body influences its ability to function properly. Osteopathic treatment aims to improve the structural organization—for example, by removing pressure from nerves—and so positively impact your health.

Treatment is based on combining these three principles. This gives osteopathy its unique philosophy and flavor. By freeing the body of disharmony, or disease, perhaps in the form of overcontracted muscles or misaligned joints, the body is better able to heal itself of a wide variety of ills.

Orthopaedic medicine

The early growth of this approach to diagnosis and treatment is largely due to the pioneering work of Dr. James Cyriax (1904–85), who trained in orthopaedics in London and subsequently practiced in the United States. He developed a system for identifying soft-tissue injuries and a non-surgical approach to their treatment.

Diagnosis The first goal of the Cyriax method is to perform an initial accurate diagnosis by thoroughly questioning and inspecting the patient, carrying out a functional examination to check for areas of pain, strengths, and weaknesses, and finally by conducting a hands-on check of the whole body.

Once a diagnosis has been made, the practitioner will need to take into account the personality of the patient, and the type, duration, and location of the problem, in order to decide on the best course of action. The Cyriax treatment options are infiltration, injection (see Prolotherapy on p.137), deep transverse massage, manipulation of the spine and extremities, mobilization, and traction. The Cyriax method is particularly effective for soft-tissue injuries.

A key component of the Cyriax treatment is transverse friction massage. This is a deep, vigorous massage applied across the muscle fibers, which activates the body's immune and self-repair systems. It stimulates the soft tissues, encouraging the breakdown of unwanted fibrous tissue and boosting normal tissue repair. The muscle fibers are eventually encouraged back into their correct position.

Chiropractic

Like osteopaths, chiropractors are primary healthcare practitioners, and they have a special interest in the impact on health made by the dysfunction of the musculo-skeletal system.

Chiropractic was discovered by Daniel D. Palmer, a magnetic healer living in Davenport, Iowa. The first chiropractic "adjustment" occurred in 1895, when Palmer restored the hearing of Harvey Lillard by manipulating his spine.

Scope of practice Most chiropractors in all countries have a similar core scope of practice, treating patients with manual manipulative techniques. American chiropractors undergo four years of full-time training. They are licensed in all states, each state having its own licensing board, with its own requirements.

Diagnosis and treatment In general, the way a chiropractor diagnoses your injury will be similar to the process used by an osteopath. In Europe, there is one difference in that chiropractors tend to make more use of X rays and are therefore more likely to have their own X-ray facilities.

Many chiropractors use a wide range of treatment modalities, while others make very extensive use of high velocity, low amplitude thrust techniques, or "adjustments." Not all chiropractors use manipulation, and some specialize, for example, in the treatment of extremities or neurological conditions.

It has often been said that chiropractors use direct short lever thrusts, applied to the joint being treated, while osteopaths utilize long levers, applying the thrusting force far from the joint being treated. In practice, many of the thrust techniques employed by both professions are very similar.

Principles Chiropractors recognize that impaired joint mobility, particularly in the spine, affects the nervous system. The aim of their treatment is to improve the alignment and mobility of joints, thus removing any distorting effect on the nervous system.

Physiotherapy

Unlike osteopaths and chiropractors, physiotherapists are not trained as primary healthcare providers. Physiotherapy is a "profession allied to medicine," and as such physiotherapists rely on medical practitioners to diagnose conditions and to prescribe physiotherapy as the treatment. However, many physiotherapists are highly skilled in the diagnosis and treatment of musculo-skeletal injuries. Physiotherapy uses physical methods, such as massage, manipulation, remedial exercise, infrared and ultraviolet rays, and heat, to promote the healing of physical injuries or disabilities. As it is more closely related to allopathic medicine, physiotherapy often takes less of a whole-body approach.

Qualifications In America, physiotherapists should be licensed by their state registration board. Training in physiotherapy typically requires three years of full-time training, leading to a bachelors degree.

Undergraduate training does not include the range of manipulative skills seen in osteopathic or chiropractic training. However, some physiotherapists undergo post-graduate training to gain such skills, and may refer to themselves as "manipulative physiotherapists" as a result.

Diagnosis and treatment As with other practitioners, physiotherapists will start by asking you about the details of how your injury occurred and the location and characteristics of your symptoms. Finding positions or movements that reproduce your symptoms is a diagnostic strategy that is frequently employed by physiotherapists.

Traditionally physiotherapists have made great use of electrotherapy modalities. These include ultrasound, interferential, lasers, and the newer infrared light therapy devices. Electrotherapy is used to produce a range of effects on tissues, such as improving blood flow, promoting inflammation, and relieving pain.

Physiotherapists often have greater experience with these tools than other types of manual therapists.

Another strong point of physiotherapy is its use of prescribed exercises for rehabilitation after injury. All of the professions utilize exercises in their treatment approaches, but physiotherapists probably do so more extensively. Practitioners from any of the professions may prescribe exercises in a very routine manner—for example, all patients with back injuries may receive the same exercises. Always ask how any prescribed exercises address your problem specifically.

Massage therapy

Undoubtedly the oldest of the manual therapies, it is not surprising that there is great diversity in the practices falling under the title of massage. Some of these approaches are used to produce the benefits of general relaxation, some are used as psychotherapeutic tools, while others specifically address musculo-skeletal symptoms and injuries.

It is important, before taking your sports injury to a massage therapist, that you check out the style of massage used. Practitioners working in gyms or health clubs are likely to deal with injuries.

The benefits of massage therapy derive from the physical changes produced, such as muscle relaxation and improved circulation, but also from the psychological effects of touch. Physical contact was perhaps one of the greatest losses in the development of modern Western medicine.

Qualifications There is a huge variation in the quality of training provided by different massage schools. Some schools provide courses specifically in "sports massage," and graduates of these courses often refer to themselves as "sports therapists." Recommendation from someone else who has been a client is often the best way to find a suitable therapist. Feel free to ask therapists about their training and their experience with problems such as yours.

Massage styles The most common basis for massage therapy in the Western world is the "Swedish massage," which has four fundamental techniques: superficial light strokes, or effleurage; deep kneading, or petrissage; rhythmic percussion, or tapotement; and deep friction. In addition to these, some massage therapists go on to train in other methods, such as muscle energy or contact and stretch techniques, along with methods for deactivating trigger points.

There are a variety of other styles of massage, some of which are traditional and others that are more modern developments. Examples of the traditional styles include:

Shiatsu comes from Japan, and utilizes pressure on acupuncture points, along with some very effective stretching and mobilization techniques. Shiatsu training in the West often involves a part-time course spanning two years or more.

Tui na (Chinese massage) is an integral part of traditional Chinese medicine, and is similar to shiatsu. Thai massage is quite vigorous. It includes some manipulative-type techniques, but these are much less specific than those used by osteopaths and chiropractors.

Rolfing is a relatively modern system of precise, deep, soft-tissue stretching techniques, used to restore the bodies structural integrity. A full course of Rolfing takes ten "sessions," but each of these sessions may take more than one treatment, depending on the degree of distortion of the individual client. Rolfing uses techniques

Massage techniques can relax tense muscles, improve circulation, and stretch tight tissues.

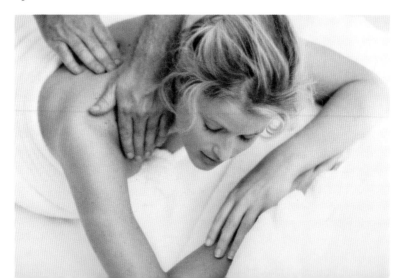

that look like massage, while producing results that are closer to one of the postural therapies (see p.132). It takes four years to train as a certified Rolfer.

Aromatherapy uses light massage to apply essential oils that have particular therapeutic purposes.

Podiatry

Nearly all sports place increased loads on the feet. Podiatrists are "foot doctors," but in addition to treating injuries to the feet, they also help restore correct function in the feet, which can have a beneficial effect on some ankle, knee, or even back injuries. It is this ability to diagnose and treat disorders in the mechanics of the feet that make podiatrists of particular value in the treatment of sports injuries. Podiatric treatment can also highly benefit injuries that occur in non-sporting contexts.

Qualifications Professional training in podiatry involves a three-year, full-time course leading to a bachelor's degree. Podiatrists can complete a further five to seven years of training in order to qualify in podiatric surgery. This increases their scope of practice to include conditions requiring surgical intervention.

Diagnosis and treatment Half of the bones in your body are in your feet. The joints are supported by ligaments and fascial tissue, and are moved and stabilized by numerous muscles. This complexity allows our feet to adapt to the wide-ranging demands caused by such complex activities as running on uneven ground.

Podiatrists examine your feet, and then often study how you walk or run. They may do this by observing or filming you on a treadmill. This process allows them to see your feet in action, so that they can diagnose any problems in your function.

Treatment often includes the use of orthotics. These are special inserts to go in your shoes, which are designed to encourage corrected function as you stand or move. Several types of insoles, or "arch support," are available to buy over the counter, but these are very different from the orthotics prescribed by a podiatrist.

Orthotics are made specifically to correct your function, after a detailed analysis of your problem, while over-the-counter supports can alter your function in inappropriate directions and even make your condition worse.

Podiatrists provide advice on footwear, helping you to choose the right shoes for you and your sport. They may also prescribe medication, carry out surgical procedures, and suggest exercises where appropriate.

Acupuncture

Treatment by inserting fine needles into the skin is an ancient art. Records suggest that acupuncture has been practiced for around five thousand years, with the earliest "needles" being made of stone.

The West has always been fascinated by acupuncture, mainly because it is so different from our familiar therapies. Yet traditionally acupuncture is not a therapy in itself, but part of Traditional Chinese Medicine, or TCM for short. TCM treatment also includes dietary modifications, the use of medicinal herbs, massage, and exercise techniques.

TCM diagnosis involves history taking and observation of the patient, with particular note being taken of the state of the tongue. Another unique element is the use of pulse diagnosis, where the characteristics of no less than six pulses are examined on each wrist.

The practitioner needs to gain an insight into the state of energy, or "Qi," imbalance in the patient, as all impairments of health are associated with energy imbalances. Treatment is then aimed at restoring balance, thus assisting the body in regaining health.

How does it work? Traditional Chinese theory maps out a network of channels, or meridians, through which energy flows throughout the body. There are specific points along the meridians where treatment influences the flow of energy, and it is into these acupuncture points that needles are inserted.

These same points may also be treated by moxibustion, whereby a small cone of dried herb is placed over the point and then lit. The herb smoulders, warming the point, and as soon as any discomfort is felt, the practitioner removes the herbs from the skin.

The main meridians are associated with different organs or qualities. For example, the large intestine meridian runs from the end of the first finger to a point near the end of the nose.

Many of these concepts are completely alien to Western anatomy and physiology, and this leads people to ridicule them initially. However, acupuncture has gained the acceptance of many doctors, simply on the strength of clinical results reported by their patients.

A major obstacle to our understanding of acupuncture is that familiar words are used, but they refer to unfamiliar concepts. When a TCM practitioner refers to the "liver," he is not talking about the physical organ, but about the "liver qualities" of a person, which may include (but not be limited to) the physical organ.

Similarly, the meridians may be referred to as channels for energy, yet no such physical channels have ever been identified by Western anatomists. However, energy does not necessarily require physical channels. You may remember seeing experiments at school where a magnet was placed under a card onto which iron filings had been sprinkled. The iron filings arranged themselves into lines, mapping out the magnetic field produced by the magnet, yet there were no physical boundaries to these energy lines.

Treatment The most surprising factor about the treatment is that it is not painful. Needles are usually inserted into several points, which are often far from the site of your injury. The practitioner may manipulate the needles, rotating them until a sense of fullness is produced at the point. The needles are then left in place, usually for several minutes. Some points that are not on a meridian may be treated if these are spontaneously tender, or "ah shi," points.

Qualifications There are a variety of different types of training, producing different types of practitioner. Some manual therapists take short courses in aspects of acupuncture, sometimes referred to as "dry needling." These courses do not cover many traditional Chinese concepts, but can still be very useful in assisting the treatment of injuries.

Western-trained TCM practitioners will typically have completed a part-time two or three year course. Most practitioners will be registered with a professional body that sets a minimum training standard. This is always worth checking.

Is it safe? Invasive procedures always raise concerns for safety, but acupuncture has a very good safety record. It is normal now for disposable needles to be used. These are pre-sterilized in sealed packs, and are disposed of after a single use, thus eliminating any risk of spreading infection.

Hydrotherapy

The therapeutic use of water has long been a significant part of the treatment provided by naturopathic physicians. A major feature that makes water so useful is its ability to deliver heat to, or draw it away from, the body.

Hydrotherapy is an ancient therapy, and one which many of us use without recognizing it. How many people have used a hot water bottle to ease pain?

Why use hydrotherapy? As mammals, we have the ability to maintain a steady internal temperature, despite variations in the temperature around us (up to a point). One of the mechanisms we use to do this is altering the distribution of our blood circulation.

When we are getting too hot, we pump more blood around our skin, so that we can dissipate heat like a radiator. That is why you get red in the face when you have been exercising vigorously indoors.

When we get cold, we do the opposite, maintaining heat by keeping more blood in our core, drawing it away from our skin. This is why people talk about "going blue in the cold." Hydrotherapy utilizes this natural mechanism, by purposefully applying heat or cold to areas of the body in order to influence the circulation.

The effects of hot and cold Warming up a part of the body opens up blood vessels, increasing the amount of blood being delivered. More blood brings more nutrients, the raw material needed to repair injuries, as well as more oxygen, which reduces the amount of scar tissue formed after an injury.

However, sustained heat can lead to the congestion of blood in the area, and this "pooling" of blood can reduce the effective circulation in the area. There is plenty of blood, but it is not moving very much, like a rush-hour gridlock where there is plenty of traffic, but nothing is flowing.

Prolonged heat can be useful in chronic injuries in tissues with poor blood supplies, such as ligaments.

Cooling an area causes the blood vessels to constrict, reducing the blood supply to that part of the body. If this is done just for a short period of time, it is followed by a reaction where the blood vessels then open wide, flushing the area with fresh blood.

Keeping an area cool for longer periods is useful when you want to reduce bleeding or prevent swelling. Reducing the blood flow makes it easier for the body to make clots to plug the damaged blood vessels. Less blood getting into the area means there is less fluid to leak out into the tissues and cause swelling.

Alternating hot and cold Once an injury has passed the stage where active bleeding is a problem, usually after about 48 hours, alternating hot and cold can increase circulation, while preventing congestion. This is also a good strategy for reducing stubborn swelling.

Apply heat first to open up the blood vessels. This brings more blood into the area, but also makes space in the veins carrying blood away from the area. Next apply cold. The blood vessels now contract and, as veins have non-return valves, the contraction pushes blood away from the area.

Each application of hot then cold causes the blood vessels to act like a tiny heart, pumping blood through the tissues. You should therefore apply hot for one minute, followed by cold for two minutes, and then repeat the whole process three to five times.

Methods Heat can be applied by immersing the injury in a bowl of hot water, wrapping it in a towel soaked in hot water, or using a commercial hot pack. The heat should not be hot enough to burn or scald.

Commercial cold packs are also available, and some of the "gel" packs can be used for hot or cold, as can "wheat bags," which are becoming increasingly popular.

A bowl of cold water with a few ice cubes in it, or a plastic bag containing water and a little ice, are other options for cold applications.

nutrition

There is increasing evidence that poor nutrition is a major contributor to many diseases, and that nutritional intervention can improve health in a wide range of conditions. Nutrition also has an important role to play in the prevention and treatment of sports injuries.

Food is a vital issue because it fuels all our activities, and provides the raw materials needed for tissue replacement and repair. The need for repair is obvious in an acute injury situation; less obvious is the ongoing repair and replacement that happens every day.

It stands to reason that if your nutrition is less than ideal, then the impaired supply of raw materials will influence the quality of tissue being rebuilt. Good nutrition is therefore an important part of preventing injuries, as it allows you to maintain strong tissues.

What is good nutrition?

Good nutrition provides all the nutrients required for optimum health, in appropriate quantities, while eliminating or minimizing the intake of toxic substances that are potentially damaging to health.

The importance of hydration

You are made up of about 70 percent water, and normal water concentrations are essential for the normal function of all systems, including your brain and muscles.

Exercise increases water loss through sweating, and replacement of this water is essential to maintaining both health and sports performance. Therefore, always drink water before, during, and after exercise.

PRINCIPLES OF GOOD NUTRITION

Nutrition is a complex subject, but three simple principles will help you to make healthy dietary choices.

- *Eat a wide variety of foods. This increases your chances of getting all the different nutrients you need, while also reducing your risk of of getting too much of any single food or nutrient. It is different foods, not just different forms of the same food, that you need. A whole wheat cereal with milk, a cheese sandwich, and a pizza are all basically wheat and milk.*
- *Minimize the processing of your food. Processing tends to remove food elements, add "non-food" elements, or distort nutrients so they no longer suit us. We have evolved with simple whole foods, and many of their synergistic combinations of nutrients suit our needs well. For example, whole grains contain carbohydrates in the form of starch, which we burn for energy. To burn carbohydrates, we need vitamin B$_1$, which is found in the husk of the grain. Remove that husk to make white flour or white rice, and we are creating a relative vitamin B$_1$ deficiency.*
- *Make sure that fresh fruit and vegetables are a staple part of your diet. They are excellent sources of many nutrients, including vitamins and minerals.*

Specific nutritional remedies

Several nutritional compounds are useful in the treatment of sports injuries.

Bromelain This enzyme, extracted from pineapple stems, increases the speed of healing of bruises and soft-tissue injuries, including bursitis. If you are taking any anti-coagulant medication to "thin your blood," check with your doctor before use.

DMSO (Dimethyl sulphoxide) & MSM (Methyl sulphonyl methane) DMSO is an industrial solvent produced as a by-product in wood pulp processing. It has a history of several decades of use in veterinary medicine for the treatment of joint injury and

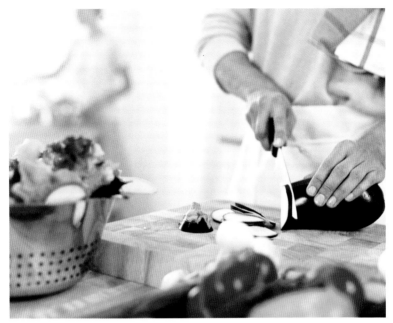

A healthy diet provides the building materials of a healthy body.

inflammation, but research on human use has been limited by lack of funding, as DMSO cannot be patented as a drug. Many people have used it for the treatment of arthritis, as it will penetrate directly through the skin, and has anti-inflammatory effects.

DMSO passing through the skin will carry other substances with it, and a new treatment combining it with the NSAID diclofenac is being researched. Contaminants on the skin, or in the DMSO, can also be carried into the body, creating a risk of poisoning. An unpleasant body and mouth odor occurs within minutes of applying DMSO to the skin, a graphic demonstration of the speed with which it passes through the skin.

Fifteen percent of absorbed DMSO is converted to MSM, which some clinicians and researchers believe is responsible for the therapeutic effects. At least some of its effect is thought to be due to its rich sulphur content.

MSM is present in many foods and is widely available as a supplement. Its recommended uses include the treatment of arthritis and soft-tissue injuries. It is not absorbed through the skin, so needs to be taken orally, and it avoids the unpleasant odor of DMSO. Clinicians suggest dosages starting at 500mg twice a day with meals, building up to 2–8g daily.

Essential fatty acids (EFAs) Your body uses chemical messengers, called prostaglandins, to turn inflammation up or down. Prostaglandins are made from dietary fats, so having the right balance of fats is important.

The diets of 90 percent of the population are low in the essential omega-3 and omega-6 fatty acids. Prostaglandins are made from dietary fats, but many people's diets are low in the essential omega-3 and omega-6 fatty acids, and prostaglandins made from these EFAs reduce inflammation. Omega-6 EFAs come from many nuts and seeds, with evening primrose oil being a popular rich source. Omega-3 EFAs are found in the oils of cold sea fish, such as mackerel and herring, and from linseed or hempseed oils.

Glucosamine sulphate This supplement is derived from the shells of shellfish. When use exceeds two weeks, it has been shown to provide better pain relief for arthritic joints than the popular NSAIDs. It has also demonstrated an effect that no drug can currently match: in a three year trial it halted the deterioration of arthritic knees. The dosage used in the trials was 1500mg a day.

Glucosamine sulphate produces considerably fewer side effects than the common anti-inflammatory drugs.

Oligomeric proanthcyanidins (OPCs) Commercially produced OPCs are usually extracted from grape seeds. They reduce the pain and swelling caused by injury or surgery.

Vitamin C and bioflavonoids These substances generally occur together in nature and provide some anti-inflammatory effect. There is some evidence that supplementing these nutrients speeds healing.

Therapeutic dosages of vitamin C vary from 500mg to several grams daily. A useful supplement will provide 500–1000mg of vitamin C, with 100–500mg of bioflavonoids.

natural
remedies

Herbs, homeopathic remedies, and essential oils can all help in the treatment of sports injuries. Many of these remedies have a long history, and are still used today because they have demonstrated effectiveness and safety.

You should, however, always consult a practitioner before using any of these remedies if you are using other medicines, or if you are pregnant or breast-feeding.

Herbs

Herbs are our oldest medicines, and are still the major medicines in many parts of the world. Many modern drugs are derived from traditional herbs. Herbs provide a complex mixture of many ingredients, and it is often this combination that results in the effectiveness and the safety of the remedy, rather than any single ingredient.

Herbs are available as freeze-dried powders, often sold in capsules, or as liquid extracts dissolved in alcohol. Always follow the manufacturer's guidance on dosage.

Aloe vera The gel from this plant supports wound healing. It is useful for treating abrasions and burns, including friction or sunburn.

Devil's claw (Harpagophytum) Extracted from the tuber of an African plant, this remedy for rheumatic pain and arthritis appears to have both anti-inflammatory and pain-relieving properties. This makes it useful in the treatment of many sports injuries, including sprains, strains, and back injuries. It is less likely to produce digestive upset than NSAIDs are.

Frankincense (Boswellia) has anti-inflammatory and pain relieving properties, and may help protect cartilage against injury. Research has demonstrated that it improves blood circulation to the joints. It is particularly indicated in the treatment of bursitis.

Ginger Ginger has potent anti-inflammatory effects. Research suggests that it is more effective than NSAIDs. Unlike these drugs, which have been put forward as causes of stomach ulcer, ginger has been used traditionally in the treatment of ulcers.

St. John's wort *(Hypericum)* Well publicized for its anti-depressant qualities, this herb is also useful in the treatment of nerve pains, such as neuralgia and sciatica. Consider it for any injury causing referred pain.

Turmeric This spice has powerful anti-inflammatory and pain-relieving properties. It has demonstrated anti-inflammatory effects at least as potent as several steroid drugs when dealing with acute inflammation. No undesirable side effects have been recorded, even with very high doses.

Turmeric is useful in the treatment of sprains and strains as well as osteo- and rheumatoid arthritis. Dosage is about one ounce of the powder daily.

Adaptogens

Several herbs help us to adapt to stressful circumstances, including sports training and competition. The term **adaptogen**, meaning supporting the ability to cope with various stressors, was initially coined with reference to **Ginseng**. The name Ginseng refers to Asian or American **Panax Ginseng**, and also to the unrelated herb Eleutherococcus, which is sometimes called "Russian or Siberian Ginseng." There is some scientific evidence that Ginseng can improve sporting performance. **Ashwagandha** is

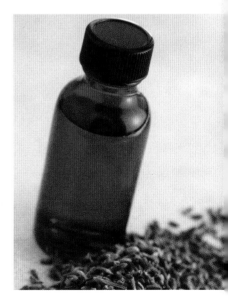

Many natural remedies have proven their effectiveness over hundreds of years.

sometimes called "Indian Ginseng" because of its similar properties. The Siberian herb **Rhodiola** is also an adaptogen, and appears to enhance physical-exercise capacity, immune function, and memory.

Homeopathic remedies

Homeopathy was developed by the German physician Samuel Hahnemann in the late eighteenth century, and is based on the principle of "treating like with like." Homeopaths use highly diluted remedies that, in their undiluted form, would cause the symptoms they are used to treat.

Homeopaths consider the more dilute the remedy, the more potent its effect. The "symptom picture" of a remedy is discovered by giving the substance to healthy volunteers, and recording the symptoms produced. Remedies are available as pills or liquids in dropper bottles for internal use, and some are available as creams for external use. The following list contains the most useful remedies for sports injuries.

Arnica This is used for the treatment of shock (involved in most injuries), trauma, bruising, and bleeding. It is often the first remedy used.

Bryonia Used for sprains and strains, byronia is used where any movement or pressure makes the symptoms worse.

Calendula This cream is applied externally for blisters, dry skin, or minor cuts.

Hypericum This is used internally for the treatment of nerve injuries or deep cuts.

Rhus tox Used for sprains, strains, and tendinosis; rhus tox is used where pain is initially aggravated by movement, but eased by continued movement.

Ruta grav This is used for sprains and strains that do not respond well to rhus tox or bryonia. It is useful after arnica for "bruises" to bone.

Symphytum This is the main remedy for the treatment of fractures. Symphytum is also useful in the treatment of eye injuries.

Essential oils

Aromatherapists use a wide range of essential oils, usually applied by massage, in the treatment of injuries. They are made up by adding just a few drops of the essential oils to a carrier oil, such as sweet almond or grape seed oil. A wide variety of "recipes" are used, combining oils to suit specific kinds of injuries.

The following oils are useful in the treatment of sports injuries. They can be applied by placing two or three drops of the essential oil in a teaspoonful of carrier oil, to make a massage oil, or by dropping 5–10 drops in your bath water just before you get in. **Essential oils are for external use only.**

Black pepper This must be used in tiny amounts. It aids the healing of joint pain, nerve pain, and muscular pain.

Ginger stimulates circulation, making it useful in the treatment of muscular pains and stiffness. It also has anti-inflammatory properties, so it treats joint injury and arthritis.

Lavender has pain-relieving and relaxing properties, making it useful for sprains, muscular aches, and stiffness. It is also beneficial for bruises, stings, and burns.

Lemon grass This has similar properties to tea tree oil (see below), with the addition of being useful in the treatment of muscular aches and pains.

Marjoram This is used in the treatment of bruises, sprains, muscular aches, and stiffness. Marjoram has pain-relieving, antiseptic, and muscle-relaxing qualities.

Rosemary has pain-relieving, relaxing, and antiseptic properties. It is used in the treatment of both muscular pain and nerve pain (neuralgia).

Tea tree This has potent anti-bacterial, anti-viral, and anti-fungal properties. It is particularly useful in the treatment of athlete's foot.

White camphor Used in the treatment of sprains, muscular pains, and stiffness. Make sure you get white camphor, as the brown or yellow versions are toxic.

postural
therapies

If you drive a car using harsh acceleration, then sudden braking, crashing the gears and bumping up on curbs when you park, you couldn't reasonably expect the car to continue running smoothly and quietly.

Like our cars, the way we use ourselves affects the way we function. Good use leads to smooth efficient movements with minimal energy wastage, decreasing stress and wear on muscles and joints, and reduced risk of injury.

Our use of our bodies also influences aspects of our general health, as poor physical use can interfere with the mechanical action of breathing, the free flow of circulation, and the normal transmission of information through your nervous system.

Our postures, or the way we use our bodies, are linked to our state of mind, influencing whether we feel happy or sad. If your posture is slumped downward, with shallow breathing, it is very hard to feel energetic or happy. One of the most immediate ways of increasing your energy level is by using breathing exercises, such as diaphragmatic breathing. These also ease tension and promote calmness. Similarly, if you stand tall and relaxed, with the crown of your head floating out of your neck and straight upward on top of a lengthened spine, depression will be diminished.

Improving body use helps us to get more enjoyment from our sport by improving our performance and reducing our chances of suffering injuries.

Where does poor use come from?

If you watch healthy young children, up to around the age of five or six, you will see excellent body use. They naturally have elegant body alignment, and move with fluid, relaxed ease. While they still lack some complicated skills—they may have difficulty catching a ball—what they can do, they do with grace and ease.

This is a clue as to how we begin to lose our natural body use; we shift our focus more onto *what* we can do, rather than *how* we do it. In our drive to succeed, we replace doing it well with "trying hard." We focus on achieving an outcome, while losing awareness of the process we are using to get there. In this way, we begin to distort the patterns of natural good use that most of us had as children. The old saying tells us that "practice makes perfect," and so the more we practice these distorted patterns of movement, the better we get at performing them.

Years down the line, we have lost awareness of what constitutes good use. We no longer realize when we are tensing ourselves unnecessarily, scrunching our bodies into distorted shapes, and limiting our scope for movement.

A familiar example is the inability of teenagers to "stand up straight." Even if they are prepared to try to stand up straight, they have often lost access to the internal reference of how to stand up in a relaxed manner without slouching.

Other sources of poor use include imitating role models with poor use (members of families often have similar patterns of use); compensating for unresolved injuries; engaging in occupations involving sustained postures or repeated movements; and repeated physical expression of mental or emotional states.

However, we can rediscover our natural sense of good use. There are a variety of approaches that allow us to regain our awareness of *how* we do and *what* we do. They enable us once again to enjoy the physical pleasure of efficient, easy movement, with all its attendant benefits.

The therapies

Any system that helps us to regain good body use will have to be more than a series of physical exercises. A key component is an increased awareness of how we actually use ourselves day by day. Without this, any exercises will be performed with our current, unconscious, poor use, thus strengthening our bad habits by practicing them more intensely.

To increase awareness, the therapies have practices that challenge us mentally as much as they do physically. Initially, the exercises will seem difficult, or at least odd, because most of us are unfamiliar with focusing our attention on how we do things.

Alexander technique This technique enables you to improve your physical and general health through better posture. An Alexander teacher observes how you use your body in your sport and everyday movements, and notes when you use it incorrectly. He or she will show you how to change harmful postures by guiding or gently manipulating your body into a more natural position.

The teacher provides both physical and verbal feedback, helping you to become aware of your patterns of unnecessary strain and effort, so that you can "inhibit" these patterns. By becoming aware of your habitual tensions, you can decide not to tense up, thus making a movement with greater ease and fluidity.

Practice allows these very conscious and purposeful improvements in use to gradually become habitual, so that improved use becomes unconscious.

Pilates Classes in pilates have recently become very popular, and are available in many gyms and leisure clubs. Pilates utilizes specific physical exercises, with detailed attention paid to how the exercises are performed. Pilates combines elements of yoga, dance, gymnastics, and Alexander technique by using controlled exercise, stretches, and breathing techniques. It targets key postural muscles to achieve physical stability and balance in the trunk by strengthening weak muscles and lengthening the short ones. Postural alignment is corrected and, as a result, joint mobility is improved. Pilates is also excellent for rehabilitation following sports injuries.

The exercises are designed to develop eight key qualities:

- Relaxation—to release inappropriate muscle tension.
- Concentration—to increase awareness of body use.
- Alignment—to develop proper use of body components.
- Breathing—to free the breath and coordinate it with movement.
- Centering—to build strength in the core stabilizing muscles.
- Coordination—to develop improved patterns of movement.
- Flowing movements—to cultivate the appropriate sequencing of muscle activity.
- Stamina—to help you sustain the other qualities.

Yoga This ancient system has evolved over several thousand years as a method of body, mind, and spiritual development. The physical component, hatha yoga, provides us with a way of enjoying many physical health benefits, whether or not we are seeking spiritual development.

Classes usually include the practice of:

- Asana—the physical postures that form the most visually recognizable aspect of yoga practice. These are divided into standing poses, forward bends, back bends, twists and inversions, and poses that involve turning upside down. In some styles of yoga, such as "Ashtanga," the poses are actually combined to produce flowing sequences.
- Pranayama—the practice of breathing exercises. The control of breathing spans conscious and unconscious mechanisms. Different patterns of breathing can significantly alter both mental and physical states.
- Relaxation—often practiced at the end of a class.

There are a variety of styles of yoga, each placing varied degrees of emphasis on relaxation, physical alignment, strength, and flexibility. Discuss with your teachers what it is you want to get out of yoga practice, to ensure that you find a class that is absolutely right for you.

Systems such as yoga can increase strength, flexibility, and body awareness, leading to improvements in body use.

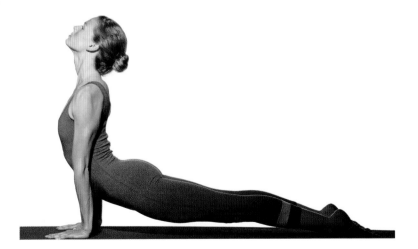

surgery

Surgery can provide several benefits in the treatment of sports injuries—namely debris removal, stabilization, repair, and reconstruction. Let's look at knee injuries as an example.

- **Debris removal** Surgeons are frequently required to remove "loose bodies," such as small fragments of cartilage or bone from inside a joint. Such fragments can cause pain, swelling, and locking of the knee.
- **Stabilization** Fractures require stability in order to heal fully. With a knee injury like osteochondritis desicans, in which a larger fragment of bone breaks off the thigh bone within the knee joint, surgical stabilization is often required.
- **Repair** Tears of the cartilage within the knee can often be repaired, depending on the location of the tear. The surgeon will remove any non-viable tissue, and will stitch (suture) the torn edges of the remaining cartilage back together.
- **Reconstruction** If the anterior cruciate ligament is completely ruptured, it can be surgically reconstructed using a slice taken from the patella (kneecap) tendon. Rapid progress is currently being made in the use of such grafting techniques.

Recent advances

The surgical treatment of sports injuries has progressed at an incredible rate over the last 30 years. Specialist sports-injury surgical units are developing more effective procedures, and gaining a better knowledge of the nature and diagnosis of injuries.

Arthroscopy This is the application of "keyhole" surgery to joints. Tiny fiber optic probes are inserted into the joint through small incisions, allowing the surgeon to view the inside of the joint on a monitor. This has huge potential in the diagnosis of joint injuries, but increasing numbers of operations are also being performed using this approach. The advantages of arthroscopic operations include less tissue healing being required, which leads to easier rehabilitation and a quicker return to activity. It is not unusual for patients to return to physical exercise in three to six weeks.

WHEN SHOULD YOU SEE A SURGEON?

Some injuries require emergency surgical attention; examples of such injuries are identified in this book by the warning boxes. In other injuries, where surgical treatment might be required, it is often best kept for times when conservative care has failed. It can be useful to get advice from both surgical and non-surgical professionals before making a decision.

Magnetic resonance imaging (MRI) scans These use powerful magnetic fields to generate detailed images of the inside of body structures. Unlike X rays, they do not use radiation, and they "see" soft tissues of the body such as muscles and ligaments in addition to bones. As injured tissues can be visualized without any invasive procedures, MRI scans are great in the diagnosis of injuries.

Prolotherapy This is gaining ground as an alternative to surgery for some injuries. It involves a series of injections of simple substances, such as sugar, often combined with a local anaesthetic, into damaged tissues. These substances act as local irritants, stimulating the tissue to proliferate, growing new tissue to repair the damaged tissue. Clinical results from doctors who utilize prolotherapy suggest that it can be used to treat a wide variety of problems, including ligament laxity in knee or ankle problems, tennis or golfer's elbow, Achilles tendon injuries, and lower back pain.

Arthroscopic surgery minimizes trauma, speeding return to normal activity.

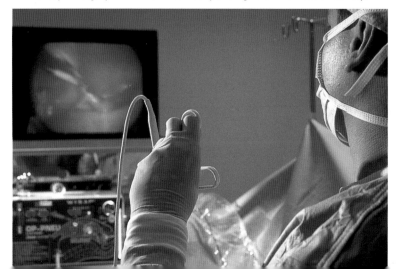

rehabilitation

This is one of the most vital, yet the most overlooked aspect of injury management among recreational athletes. Once acute symptoms have eased, most of us jump right back into the game. This is why we end up reinjured.

An injury means that at least one of our tissues was unable to cope with the stresses of our sport. A key to the safe use of exercises during rehabilitation is that they should be pain-free during performance, and they should not cause an increase in symptoms afterward. At the early stage of tissue healing, the tissue is being built and is not very strong. Overly vigorous exercises will tear down the newly repaired tissue, taking you back to square one. Just resting the injury is not useful either—the resulting healed tissues will not be able to withstand the stresses imposed by normal use.

Progressive exercises place gradually increasing loads on the tissue, so it organizes its structure to withstand those loads. Exercises must always be performed within pain-free limits.

Building strength

Exercises that strengthen muscles also strengthen tendons. This is clearly necessary with muscle or tendon injuries, but it also has benefits in rehabilitating other tissues. Building strength in muscles that stabilize a joint reduces the strain imposed on the ligaments of that joint. This is why exercises to strengthen thigh muscles are used in the rehabilitation of knee ligament injuries, for example.

You need to identify which muscles need strengthening, both to rehabilitate the injury and increase your ability to withstand the loads of your activity. It is best to combine exercises that target the injured tissues with a general program of exercises to improve overall strength. Muscle imbalance makes injuries more likely, so ensuring a balanced development of strength helps to prevent any problems in the future.

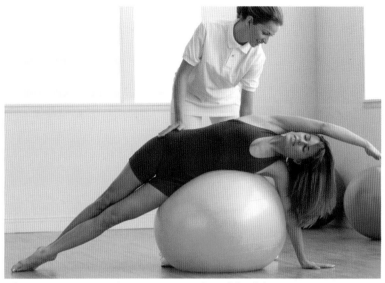

After an injury, it is vital to restore strength and flexibility to prevent reinjury.

Increasing flexibility

Stretching exercises, performed within pain-free limits, encourage repairing fibers to line up to withstand the tensile strain on the tissue. This results in tissues that are adapted to cope with functional stresses. If tissues are left stiff after an injury not only are they more liable to tear again, but they also interfere with normal movement.

Functional exercises

These are designed to restore skilled coordination. Rehabilitating a knee injury might involve jogging, progressing to running in straight lines, running with diagonal changes of direction, and so on. Pain indicates that you have tried to progress too fast and that you should go back a couple of steps in the program.

Maintaining fitness

Keeping fit will speed your recovery, and make rehabilitation quicker and easier. Find an activity that maintains fitness without aggravating your injury. For example, the squash player with "tennis elbow" can still run, the soccer player with the twisted knee can try a stationary bike, and the runner with Achilles bursitis can swim.

glossary

Abrasion—skin damaged by friction, a graze

Acute—a condition which is short term, or a symptom which is sharp or sudden

Aerobic exercise—moderate intensity exercise in which the heart and lungs can supply all the oxygen needed by the muscles

Altered sensation—a change in normal skin sensation, including "pins and needles," tingling, and numbness

Anaerobic exercise—high intensity exercise in which the muscles need for oxygen is not met by the heart and lungs

Arthroscopy—examining the inside of a joint using a fiber optic probe

Avulsion fracture—an injury where a tendon or ligament pulls off a piece of bone

Bruise—bleeding that occurs under the skin

Bursa—a fluid filled sack which acts as a cushion between tissues

Chronic—a condition that persists over a long period of time

Clavicle—collarbone

Contusion—a bruise

CPR—cardiopulmonary resuscitation, the first aid treatment used when breathing and the heart have stopped

Dislocation—an injury where the bones of a joint are separated abnormally

EFAs—essential fatty acids, components of fat which are essential for survival and health. EFA deficiencies influence inflammation and healing.

Fracture—injury involving damage to a bone

Haematoma—a pooling of blood in the tissues

Iliotibial band—strong band of connective tissue running down the outside of the thigh

Inflammation—the first stage of the healing process. Signs of inflammation are redness, heat swelling, and pain.

Joint dysfunction—a restriction of normal joint movement that is reversible

Laceration—a sharp cut

Lateral—relating to the outer side of the body, away from the midline

Lymph—the fluid which leaks out of blood vessels to carry nutrients to the cells of the body. Lymph is then collected in lymphatic vessels.

Medial—relating to the inner side of the body, toward the midline

MRI—magnetic resonance imaging, a scan that produces pictures of body tissues, including muscles, ligaments, and nerves.

NSAIDs—non-steroidal anti-inflammatory drugs. A family of pain relieving drugs, including aspirin, ibuprophen, naproxen, and diclofenac, frequently employed in the treatment of sports injuries.

Patella—kneecap

RICE—stands for Rest, Ice, Compression, and Elevation, the first response to all soft tissue injuries

Sacroiliac joint—paired joints at the back of the pelvis

Scapula—shoulder blade

Sprain—injury involving tearing of fibers of a ligament or joint capsule

Sternum—breastbone

Strain—injury involving tearing of fibers of a muscle

Symphysis pubis—joint at the front of the pelvis

Synovial fluid—lubricating fluid produced by the lining of joints

Ultrasound—high frequency sound that can be used diagnostically (ultrasound scan) and as a therapy to stimulate inflammation and healing

Warm-up—preparing the body for exercise by increasing the temperature of and circulation to muscles

organizations

Acupuncture
American Academy of Medical Acupuncture
5820 Wilshire Blvd., Suite 500
Los Angeles, CA 90036
Telephone: (213) 937-5514
www.medicalacupuncture.org

Alexander Technique
North American Society of Teachers of the
Alexander Technique
3010 Hennepin Ave. South, Suite 10
Minneapolis, MN 55408
Telephone: (612) 824-5066
www.sportstherapy.com/alexan.htm

Aromatherapy
National Association for Holistic Aromatherapy
4509 Interlake Ave. N., #233
Seattle, WA 98103-6773
Telephone: (206) 547-2164
www.naha.org

Chiropractic
American Chiropractic Association
1701 Clarendon Blvd.
Arlington, VA 22209
Telephone: (800) 986-4636
www.amerchiro.org

Herbal Medicine
American Herbalists Guild
P.O. Box 1683
Soquel, CA 95073
Telephone: (408) 464-2441
www.americanherbalistsguild.com

Homeopathy
National Centre for Homeopathy
801 North Fairfax St., Suite 306
Alexandria, VA 22314
Telephone: (703) 548-7790
www.homeopathic.org

Massage
American Massage Therapy Association
820 Davis Street, Suite 100
Evanston, IL 60201-4444
Telephone: (708) 864-0123
www.amtamassage.org

Naturopathy
American Association of Naturopathic
Physicians
P.O. Box 20386
Seattle, WA 98102
Telephone: (206) 323-7610
www.naturopathic.org

Nutrition
American Academy of Sports Dieticians and
Nutritionists
P.O. Box 4073
East Dedham, MA 02075
Telephone: (617) 817-0804
www.aasdn.org

Osteopathy
American Academy of Osteopathy
3500 DePauw Blvd., Suite 1080
Indianapolis, IN 46268-1136
Telephone: (317) 879-0563
www.academyofosteopathy.org

American Osteopathic Association
142 East Ontario St.
Chicago, IL 60611
Telephone: (312) 280-5800
www.aoa-net.org

Physiotherapy
American Physical Therapy Association
1111 North Fairfax St.
Alexandria, VA 22314-1488
Telephone: (703) 684-2782
www.apta.org

Podiatry
American Podiatric Medical Association
9312 Old Georgetown Rd.
Bethesda, MD 20814
Telephone: (301) 571-9200
www.apma.org

Yoga
Yoga Journal
2054 University Ave., Suite 600
Berkeley, CA 94704
Telephone: (951) 841-9200
www.yogajournal.com

index